Choosing General Practice

Choosing General Practice

Your Career Guide

Edited by

Anne Hastie
Department of Postgraduate General Practice Education
London Deanery, UK

Anne Stephenson
Department of General Practice and Primary Care
King's College London, UK

Blackwell
Publishing

BMJ|Books

© 2008 by Blackwell Publishing
BMJ Books is an imprint of the BMJ Publishing Group Limited, used under licence

Blackwell Publishing, Inc., 350 Main Street, Malden, Massachusetts 02148-5020, USA
Blackwell Publishing Ltd, 9600 Garsington Road, Oxford OX4 2DQ, UK
Blackwell Publishing Asia Pty Ltd, 550 Swanston Street, Carlton, Victoria 3053, Australia

First published 2008

1   2008

Library of Congress Cataloging-in-Publication Data

Choosing general practice : your career guide / edited by Anne Hastie, Anne Stephenson.
   p. ; cm.
Include index.
ISBN: 978-1-4051-7070-3 (pbk. : alk. paper)
1. Physicians (General practice)–Vocational guidance–Great Britain.   2. Medicine–Vocational
guidance–Great Britain.   I. Hastie, Anne.   II. Stephenson, Anne.
   [DNLM: 1. Family Practice–Great Britain. 2. Vocational Guidance–Great Britain. W89 C548 2008]
   R729.5.G4C48 2008
   610.71′143–dc22
                                        2007028574
ISBN: 978-1-4051-7070-3

A catalogue record for this title is available from the British Library

Set in 9.5/12pt Minion by Aptara Inc., New Delhi, India

Commissioning Editor: Mary Banks
Development Editors: Lauren Brindley and Victoria Pittman
Production Controller: Rachel Edwards

For further information on Blackwell Publishing, visit our website:
http://www.blackwellpublishing.com

Contents

Contributors

Nav Chana, MA Ed, FRCGP
Associate Director
Department of Postgraduate General Practice Education
London Deanery

Maria Elliott, D'Obn, RCOG, MMEd
Honorary Senior Lecturer
Department of General Practice and Primary Care
King's College London

Helen Graham, DCH, FRCGP, FHEA
Senior Lecturer in General Practice and Primary Care
Division of Medical Education
King's College London

Anne Hastie, MBE MSc, DRCOG, FRCGP FHEA
Director
Department of Postgraduate General Practice Education
London Deanery

Neil Jackson, FRCGP, DRCOG, DFFP, FHEA
Dean of Postgraduate General Practice
London Deanery

Catherine Jenson, MA, DRCOG, DCH, MRCGP
General Practice Tutor and Sessional General Practitioner
Broomwood Road Surgery
Kent

Roger Jones, MA, DM, FRCP, FRCGP, FMedSci, FFPHM, FHEA
Head
Department of General Practice and Primary Care
King's College London

Anwar Ali Khan, FRCGP
Associate Director
Department of Postgraduate General Practice Education
London Deanery

Roger May, MBE, FRCGP
General Practitioner (retired)

Steve Mowle, FRCGP, DFFP, DipMedEd
Associate Director
Department of Postgraduate General Practice Education
London Deanery

Amanda Platts, FRCGP, FRCP
Associate Director
Department of Postgraduate General Practice Education
London Deanery

John Rees, MD, FRCP
Professor of Medical Education
King's College London

Richard Savage, MSc, FRCGP
Programme Director
Guys & St. Thomas Hospital VTS
Chair
South London Organisation of Vocational Training Schemes

Suzanne Savage, FRCCP
Associate Director
Department of Postgraduate General Practice Education
London Deanery

John Spicer, FRCGP, FHEA, MA, DFFP
Tutor in Clinical Law & Ethics
St George's
University of London

Anne Stephenson, MBChB, Dip. Obst., PhD (Med), FHEA
Director of Community Education
Department of General Practice and Primary Care
King's College London

Tim Swanwick, MA, FRCGP, MA Ed
Director
Department of Postgraduate General Practice Education
London Deanery

Rebecca Viney, MRCGP, DipAD, FHEA, DipOccMed
Associate Director
Department of Postgraduate General Practice Education
London Deanery

Jan Welch, MBE, FRCP, FFFLM
Director
South East Thames Foundation School
Guy's Hospital
London

Julia Whiteman, MA, MRCGP, PRCOG
Deputy GP Director
Department of Postgraduate General Practice Education
London Deanery

Foreword

General practice and primary care are now at the forefront of health provision and health policy thinking in the United Kingdom. The recognition of the importance of the 'benign gatekeeper' role of the generalist clinician in the National Health Service (NHS), which is associated with high-quality and cost-effective care, led some years ago to the concept of a Primary Care Led NHS and, more recently, to an even clearer policy direction towards supporting more community-based medical services. The introduction of the Quality Outcomes Framework (QoF) as part of the GP contract, combined with a reduction of the pressures to provide out-of-hours and emergency care, has meant that general practice now represents a career choice which can be both professionally and financially rewarding. Lingering concerns remain, however, about a drift away from some of the core values of general practice, which include personal continuity of care, 24-hour responsibility for patients and a commitment to domiciliary care and home visiting.

This career guide to general practice not only takes the reader on a fascinating journey from medical school, through undergraduate teaching and postgraduate training, to a post as a principal in general practice, but, more importantly, emphasises the wide range of opportunities that open up to general practitioners (GPs) after postgraduate qualification. While, for most GPs, contact with individual patients and the care of the practice population will remain at the centre of their professional lives, there is scope to create a rich professional life involving undergraduate teaching, postgraduate training, research, the development of special clinical interests and a range of management and leadership roles.

About half of all medical graduates will become GPs. General practice now contributes to approaching 15% of the undergraduate medical curriculum, and medical students often have their first experience of a GP's surgery within a few weeks of entering medical school. John Rees, who directs undergraduate medical education at King's College London School of Medicine, explains how to prepare for application and admission to medical school, and the undergraduate teaching programme, with its emphasis on patient contact, one-to-one instruction, the acquisition of interpersonal and communication skills and the delivery of high-quality clinical care, is described by Helen Graham, who leads on quality assurance at KCL. The complexities of the newly established Foundation Programmes, which lead on to specialist training, and specialist training itself, follow, and Nav Chana describes the pivotal role that the Royal College of General Practitioners has played in setting standards for clinical care and for professionalism in our discipline.

In subsequent chapters post-vocational training, flexible working and returner and retainer schemes are described in detail, and Rebecca Viney and Catherine Jenson explain the intricacies of becoming a principal, a partner or a salaried GP. Maria Elliott describes how a variety of roles in general practice can be combined into a satisfying portfolio of activities, which are designed to ensure continuing stimulation, challenge and job satisfaction. General practitioners who have already acquired special skills during their hospital training, or who wish to develop knowledge and expertise in particular clinical areas, are able to join the GPwSI (General Practitioners with Special Interests) scheme, in which GPs work in a range of clinical areas, providing additional expertise, intermediate care and service development advice to local practices and to primary care trusts (PCTs). We also cover professional values, leadership and management and even provide guidance on approaching retirement from clinical practice.

My own perspective is that of an academic general practitioner who turned to research and teaching after working for several years as an NHS general practitioner in a country town in the south of England. A quarter of a century ago we lacked an evidence base for practice that was derived from practice-based research, and depended on the results of studies undertaken by hospital specialists. Over the last 25 years research in general practice has transformed our understanding of the consultation, patients' behaviour, diagnostic method, chronic disease management and health promotion, so that we are now able to refer to research undertaken in and on general practice to inform our clinical decision making and long-term management of patients. There is still much to do and, in a changing NHS, constant re-evaluation of service provision and therapeutic interventions will be needed to chart a course through an increasingly complex medical landscape.

We hope that this book will appeal to readers at every stage of the general practice journey. We would like to think that it will wet the appetites of those at an early stage in their medical careers, who perhaps have not understood that general practice involves more than seeing patients in surgeries and dealing with everyday medical and psychosocial problems. We should not forget that most patients with serious illness usually see their GP first, so that general practitioners need to be expert in the management of serious, life-threatening disorders as well as being adept in providing reassurance and support for minor, self-limiting disorders and life difficulties. One welcome feature of the new Foundation Years Scheme is that over half of all postgraduate doctors will spend 4 months in general practice. This may be just as important, if not more so, for doctors who end up as specialists than for those who become GPs, and we hope that this volume will provide some landmarks for those who are uncertain about their next career move. Whenever a specialist registrar has joined me in my surgery the invariable response has been surprise at the variety of problems presented by the patients they have seen, and an appreciation of the broad range of expertise that a GP requires to provide satisfactory first-contact care to them.

We also hope that GPs who are becoming established in practice will find something of value in this book. Notwithstanding the satisfaction of providing personal and continuing care to a patient population, the opportunity for professional refreshment afforded by taking time out to pursue a different aspect of general practice should not be underestimated.

Anne Hastie and Anne Stephenson are to be congratulated on marshalling an excellent cast of contributors to this book, which deserves wide readership and which, as far as I know for the first time, describes the rich professional world into which a career in general practice can lead.

Roger Jones
King's College London

Preface

The editors of this book, as well as the authors of the chapters, have a passion for general practice and have spent a lot of time throughout their careers guiding and training potential general practitioners (GPs) as well as supporting those already in practice. Medicine is an art as much as a science and this is particularly true of general practice. The holistic and long-term approach to patients and their families and communities makes general practice a rewarding and satisfying career. Working as part of the general practice and primary care team and being involved in teaching and research provides the support and stimulation that militates against professional isolation and burnout and promotes professional development and life-long learning. An appropriately trained general practitioner brings skills that are crucial in managing patients in primary care. Good GPs have the ability to manage patients with complex problems and co-morbidities. They can manage uncertainty and risk, which helps reduce hospital utilisation and its additional costs.

Medicine as a career has seen many changes in recent decades for a variety of reasons, some driven by the profession while others by government initiatives as well as external factors. General practice training is not as long as other specialties and the lifetime earnings of general practitioners are relatively higher than those of many hospital colleagues. However, it still takes at least 10 years to train as a general practitioner, which includes 5 or 6 years as an undergraduate (as few as four if on a graduate entry programme), 2 years of foundation training and 3 years of specialty training.

Undergraduate medical education in the United Kingdom has gone through a period of rapid change since the 1993 General Medical Council Report *Tomorrow's Doctors*.[1] As a result of this report there has been a reduction in factual learning, more experience in a variety of clinical settings, a greater integration of basic medical science and clinical practice and an increasing focus on professional development. Medical educators have been required to encourage and support students' self-directed learning and provide greater supervision and more careful assessment of student learning and development. At the same time a reduction in the number and length of hospital stays for patients has reduced the opportunities for undergraduate teaching in hospital settings. A large number of general practitioners keen to teach students, often highly trained as educators of GP registrars, as well as the wealth of learning opportunities in the community has meant that an increase in undergraduate placements in general practice has been a natural development. Medical students value the small-group and high-quality teaching that they receive from general practitioners and primary care teams as well as the opportunities to learn about health promotion and the management of people with common illnesses. In 2001, UK academic Departments of General Practice and Primary Care contributed an average of 9% of all teaching in undergraduate medical curricula[2] and this has increased to 13% in 2006 (paper in progress).

In 2003 the Department of Health[3] first published details of Modernising Medical Careers (MMC) in response to a proposal from the Chief Medical Officer to review the house officer grade.[4] This has resulted in a reorganisation of postgraduate training for doctors with the following main changes.

- The introduction of a 2-year foundation programme to replace the pre-registration House Officer (PRHO) and first Senior House Officer (SHO) years.
- The development of a 'run-through' grade for specialty training, including general practice. MMC has created the opportunity to improve general practice training, making it more flexible and competency based.

The curriculum for postgraduate general practice training is competency based with an emphasis on learning in the workplace, supervision and assessment. The curriculum covers the core GP skills,[5] which are:

- Primary care management
- Person-centred care
- Specific GP problem-solving skills
- Comprehensive approach
- Community orientation
- Holistic approach.

The Postgraduate Medical Education and Training Board (PMETB) took over the statutory responsibility for approving postgraduate medical education and training for general practice from the Joint Committee on Postgraduate Training for General Practice (JCPTGP) on 30 September 2005. New regulations will allow PMETB to be more flexible in the type of training and experience that can be approved in order to allow doctors to be eligible to become a GP.

Learning doesn't stop at the end of undergraduate courses and GP training and all GPs are involved in their continuing professional development (CPD).

General practice is increasingly becoming a first choice of career for new doctors and the introduction of placements in general practice during foundation programmes is expected to attract more doctors into general practice.

The number of women working in medicine has increased every decade since the introduction of the National Health Service (NHS) in 1948 and it is predicted that women doctors will outnumber men by 2012.[6] Men and women are seeking a better work life balance and the demand for part-time and flexible ways of training and working has been turned into an increasing reality. This has been supported and encouraged by the Department of Health through their Improving Working Lives initiative.[7] The traditional model of GPs who work full-time in one practice for their working career is outdated. Part-time clinical responsibilities combined with teaching, research, developing special clinical interests or simply achieving an appropriate work/life balance are becoming the norm.

In 2004 a new contract for general practice was introduced,[8] which replaced the previous 1990 contract. General practitioners are now paid for essential (core) services and quality care for chronic disease. Practices receive a global sum, which represents practice income and not individual GP's income as was the case under the 1990 contract. This enables practices to be more flexible in the way GPs are employed in their practice e.g. self-employed partners or salaried GPs. As a result there are increasing numbers of GPs working in salaried posts, many of who are part-time. In addition, practices can contract to provide enhanced services, which are negotiated locally. This includes the development of practitioners with special interest (GPwSI), which has enabled GPs who have developed additional skills to be paid for providing their expertise. Doctors who initially plan a hospital career sometimes decide to change to general practice for a variety of reasons. If they have several years of experience in a hospital specialty the time will not be wasted as their skills can be transferred to general practice, where they can become a GPwSI. Skills in specialties such as dermatology, cardiology, gynaecology and surgery are particularly attractive to practices and can generate additional practice income.

The importance of career counselling before choosing to enter medical training and throughout undergraduate and postgraduate training has been increasingly acknowledged, although many doctors still make career decisions by a process of elimination.[9] Counselling also needs to be available throughout GPs' working careers and into retirement to enable them to achieve their ambitions and maximum potential.

So what is the future of general practice? As the Future of General Practice Working Group said in 2004,

The future GP, at the heart of a thriving multidisciplinary team, will be a clinician and a medical generalist, with continuing important roles as gatekeeper, and as an advocate for patients. GPs have a unique constellation of skills, and their ability to deal with risk and uncertainty is central to the effectiveness of the NHS. The GP is much more than a doctor who happens to work in primary care. The medical generalist has specific skills, which will become increasingly important as society becomes progressively more technical and depersonalised.[10]

Anne Hastie and Anne Stephenson

References

1 General Medical Council (2003) *Tomorrow's Doctors. Recommendations on Undergraduate Medical Education.* London: General Medical Council.
2 Society of Academic Primary Care (2002) *Mackenzie 2 Report: New Centuries, New Challenges.* Available at http://www.sapc.ac.uk
3 Department of Health (2003) *The Response of the Four UK Health Ministers to the Consultation on Unfinished Business: Proposals for Reform of the House Officer Grade.* London: Department of Health.
4 Sir Liam Donaldson, CMO (2002) *Unfinished Business: Proposals for Reform of the House Officer Grade.* London: Department of Health.
5 Deighan M, Field S (2005) *Specialist Training for General Practice Newsletter: A Guide to the New GP Curriculum.* London: RCGP.
6 Griffiths E (2003) Just who are tomorrow's doctors? *BMJ Careers* **326**: 4.
7 Department of Health (2001) *Improving Working Lives Standard.* London: Department of Health.
8 British Medical Association (2003) *New GMS Contract 2003: Investing in General Practice.* London: BMA Publications.
9 Lambert TW, Davidson JM, Evans J, et al. (2003) Doctors' reasons for rejecting initial choice of specialties as long-term careers. *Medical Education* **37**: 312–318.
10 Royal College of General Practitioners (2004) *The Future of General Practice. A Statement by the Royal College of General Practitioners.* Available at http://www.rcgp.org.uk

Chapter 1 **General practice: past, present and future**

Roger Jones

Early days

The term 'general practitioner' was probably first used shortly after the passage of the Apothecaries Act of 1815. This was a time which marked the end of the Napoleonic Wars at the Battle of Waterloo, the invention of the stethoscope by Rene Laennec in 1816 and the flowering of the geniuses of Constable, Blake, Keats and Turner. It was also a time of unregulated medicine, when body snatching was still rife and when the medical landscape was dominated by the powerful Royal Colleges of Surgeons and Physicians. Over the next two decades, the golden age of medicine, Thomas Hodgkin, Richard Bright and Thomas Addison, all working at Guy's, made their astonishing landmark contributions. By 1844 general practitioners (GPs) had identified themselves as a well-defined section of the medical community, and attempted to form the ill-fated Association of General Practitioners.

The origins of general practice, however, can be traced far further back in medical history. The apothecaries emerged from the pepperers and spicers of the middle ages, and were originally members of the Grocer's Company of London, founded in 1373. The Worshipful Company of Apothecaries received its charter from King James in 1617, and established an apprenticeship system of training. Whilst physicians were university educated and steeped in Hippocrates and Galen, the apothecaries were involved in making and dispensing drugs prescribed by physicians; they were not allowed to diagnose or prescribe treatment.

The medical profession was decimated by the Great Plague in 1665 and the Apothecaries' Hall was destroyed in the Great Fire of London during the following year. Over the next 50 years professional tensions developed between apothecaries and physicians, and patients began to address both of

Choosing General Practice: Your Career Guide. Edited by Anne Hastie and Anne Stephenson. © 2008 Blackwell Publishing, ISBN: 978-1-4501-7070-3.

them as 'doctor', finding it difficult to distinguish between them. The physicians, fearing for the erosion of their professional status and their incomes by these medical upstarts, attempted to introduce legislation to prevent apothecaries from becoming involved in the treatment of patients, but met their own Waterloo in 1701 in the 'Rose Case', which changed the course of medical history.

The Rose Case

William Rose was an apothecary and a liveryman, practicing in St Martin's in the Fields, London. At the turn of the century he treated William Seale, a butcher in Hungerford Market, providing medication for which Seale was charged the enormous sum of £50. Seale commented that he was 'never the better but much worse' for his treatment, and complained to the Royal College of Physicians, who undoubtedly regarded this complaint as an opportunity for an important test case. The college's case against Rose was based on an act passed during the reign of Henry VIII and was brought before the Court of the Queen's Bench under the Lord Chief Justice and a jury. Rose had administered 'boluses, electuaries and juleps' without licence from the college and without direction by a physician. Because apothecaries were not allowed to 'practice physic', Rose was found guilty, but the Attorney General advised the Society of Apothecaries that they should bring a Writ of Error to the House of Lords; the case was heard in the Lords in 1704, and the original judgement was quashed. Seale's counsel, Samuel Dodd, claimed that the judgement would not only ruin Rose but all apothecaries, and that the physicians were making use of an outdated act of Parliament whose application would 'oppress the poor and be extremely prejudicial to sick persons in the case of sudden accidents or illness'. Their lordships were also aware that many physicians 'would not attend when at dinner or abed', and ruled that apothecaries could, in future, treat all illnesses, whether slight or grave.

The apothecaries

Over the next century the apothecaries widened their medical repertoire, dealing with surgical problems including abscesses, ulcers, eye diseases and toothache, and in 1740 became involved in midwifery as well, recognising that if they were able to 'deliver the babies, you will have the family as patients for life'. The Apothecaries Act of 1815 gave the Society the powers to examine and license apothecaries after serving a 5-year apprenticeship and also to carry out quality-control checks on their premises. Further regulation of prescribing and practice was introduced by the Pharmacy Act of 1852 and the Medical Act

Table 1.1 Milestones in the development of general practice: the first five hundred years

Period	Milestone
14th century	Grocers, pepperers and spicers
15th–17th century	Unregulated apothecaries, surgeons and physicians
1617	Worshipful Company of Apothecaries established by Royal Charter
1701	The Rose Case
1815	Apothecaries Act
1844	Association of General Practitioners proposed but never established
1852	Pharmacy Act
1858	Medical Act, outlawing quackery and introducing formal training and examinations

of 1858, which outlawed quackery and introduced a formal system of medical education, examination and licensing (see Table 1.1).

In the mid-nineteenth century, the future of general practice, which was by then established as a separate section of the medical profession, might have been altered for ever if the foundation of the Association of General Practitioners had been successful, and had been able to act as a professional base and political lobby for its members. Sensing competition, however, the powerful Royal Colleges, notably the Surgeons, did all they could to suppress the foundation of the Association, and contemporary accounts of the acrimonious debates which ensued make today's jibes about arrogant hospital consultants and golf-playing GPs look distinctly insipid. However, the Surgeons prevailed, and the Association of General Practitioners was stillborn. The future of general practice was further threatened by a change in the public's health care seeking behaviour. There was an extraordinary rise in the number of patients seeking first-contact care in hospital casualty departments. The records of the London Hospital, Whitechapel show that the annual number of new outpatient attendances in the early 1820s was around 5000, rising to 52,000 in the 1870s and, by 1910, had risen to 221,781. The reasons for the popularity of hospital departments as primary care providers are not clear, but this change in patient behaviour resulted in the bankruptcy of many general practitioners, who demanded that in future hospitals would only see patients who had been sent there by general practitioners with an accompanying letter. This episode marked the beginning of the referral system in the United Kingdom, and of the gatekeeper role of the general practitioner in today's National Health Service (NHS).

The beginnings of the NHS

Another central feature of the NHS, that of registration and capitation, has its roots in the National Health Insurance Act of 1911, which entitled employees earning less than £160 per year to free medical care from general practitioners taking part in the scheme, who were paid on the basis of capitation, i.e. the number of patients on their registered list or 'panel'.

The NHS was created by the National Health Service Act of 1948, a political leap of faith of great imagination and altruism, championed by the 'Welsh Wizard' Aneurin Bevan, and all the more extraordinary for emerging from the years of austerity following the Second World War. The NHS was the first, and for many years the only, health care system for which the State took responsibility, providing care free at the point of delivery irrespective of a patient's ability to pay. It encapsulated the registration system of the entire population with general practitioners and the capitation system of payment. It led to a sharper division than ever between primary care (general practice) and secondary care (hospital medicine) and confirmed the central role of the referral system from GPs to specialists. It also introduced general practitioners' 24-hour responsibility for providing care to their patients and located the responsibilities for medical education and research firmly in the hospital sector.

In a salutary counterweight to the optimism of the NHS Act, Joseph Collings published 'General Practice in England Today: A Reconnaissance' in *The Lancet* of 1950, as a result of visiting many practices around Britain. Collings commented that 'few skilled craftsmen, be they plumbers, butchers or motor mechanics, would be prepared to work under such conditions or with equipment so bad'. Irvine Loudon, our most distinguished chronicler of the history of general practice, commented:

> Just at the time when the hospital service was beginning to forge
> ahead in a state of high optimism as a result of the therapeutic
> revolution, general practice was stagnant. Post-graduate education
> was virtually non existent. All too often general practitioners, who
> were poorly paid, lacked self respect and showed little or no ambition
> to improve either their standards of practice or knowledge.

Loudon describes the change in general practice, accompanied by a rise in standards and morale, 'amounting to a transformation of general practice between 1948 and the mid-1960s', as little less than astonishing. Key factors in bringing about this sea change in professional practice and attitudes included the Family Doctors Charter of 1966 and, perhaps, most important of all, the

Table 1.2 Milestones in the development of general practice: modern times

Period	Milestone
1911	National Health Insurance Act: the origin of the 'list' system
1948	National Health Service Act: registration with GPs, services free at the point of care
1950	Collings Report, critical of infrastructure and professional standing of GPs
1952	College of General Practitioners founded
1966	Family Doctors Charter
1972	RCGP obtains its Royal Charter. Mandatory vocational training requirements for all new GPs
1991–1997	Margaret Thatcher's Internal NHS Market and GP Fundholding
2000	NHS Plan
2005	Our Health, Our Care, Our Say: re-introduction of competition and private service provision in the NHS

foundation of the College of General Practitioners, later the RCGP, at around the same time (see Table 1.2).

Modern general practice

The transformation of general practice has continued, and in many ways accelerated, over the last 40 years. Vocational training for general practice, the 3-year period of hospital and general practice-based education now mandatory for all entrants to general practice, has led the way internationally, and the standards of postgraduate education in general practice were the benchmark for the quality of training in the medical specialities for many years. Group practice, with general practitioners working alongside the other members of the primary healthcare team, has supported a system of primary care which has become the envy of the world. The increasing sophistication and widespread application of computer systems in general practice, coupled with the patient registration system, has supported high-quality clinical record keeping, audit and health promotion, as well as providing an internationally envied resource for clinical and health services research.

The growth of the academic departments of general practice in the universities has been little short of astonishing, with undergraduate teaching in general practice and community settings now accounting for up to 15% of clinical curricula, and the research output of many of these departments now bears comparison with the best primary care, clinical and health services research in the world. Despite repeated NHS reforms, the ability of general practice to provide comprehensive, continuing, personal and coordinated care to the population remains unrivalled on the international stage, and the recently introduced contractual arrangements for general practitioners have, at last, linked remuneration to the achievement of specified quality outcomes for the management of a range of important clinical conditions, encapsulated in the Quality Outcomes Framework.

The benign gatekeeper role of general practitioners, enshrined in the referrals system, has contributed significantly to the cost-effectiveness of the NHS, and the crucial importance of extending high-quality community-based care has been a central feature of Government policy, including the concept of the 'primary care-led NHS and the most recent Government White Paper, 'Our Health, Our Care, Our Say', which confirms this policy direction. Practice-Based Commissioning provides further opportunities for practices and clusters of practices to engage meaningfully in the commissioning of services that are most appropriate for particular patient populations and sub-groups.

Current concerns

In many ways general practice has been, and still remains, the jewel in the crown of the NHS, but the future is, as always, uncertain. Improvements in recruitment and retention, and in clinical standards and in the remuneration of general practitioners, have come at a price. The new contractual arrangements have signalled a retreat from 24-hour responsibility for patients, with out-of-hours care being frequently delegated to co-operatives of general practitioners, and the move from a 'small business' model of partnership working to a service in which part-time and salaried doctors play an increasingly important role, has resulted, inevitably, in an erosion of personal continuity of care, although organisational continuity is a reality in well-organised group practices. The numerous government initiatives to increase patient choice and to improve access, including NHS Direct, walk-in centres and the opportunities for non-NHS providers to deliver primary care services, are likely to create new challenges for the provision of personal, comprehensive and continuous care, recognising that ready access and convenience are priorities for many patients in an increasingly consumer-driven environment.

As doctors in primary and secondary care find themselves acting out roles that were written for them almost 700 years ago, there has never been a more exciting time to be involved in the drama of general practice and primary care in the United Kingdom. For many of us what is at stake is nothing less than the future of an extraordinary medical service which sprang from the imagination of a few visionary men in the middle of the twentieth century. For all of us there is the challenge of providing the best possible care to our population in the twenty-first century.

A vision of the future

How might general practice look in 20, 50 and 100 years' time? Whilst much foreseeable change will be driven by technological advances, globalisation and changing demography, the emergency of new infectious diseases and the burden of the chronic, non-communicable disease will all play their part. Much change will be unimaginable at the present time.

We will undoubtedly know much more about our bodies in health and disease in a decade's time, as genomics becomes more sophisticated and more affordable and the sequencing of our genes begins to fulfil the promise of the revolution started by Crick and Watson. Our ability to give accurate prognoses will be severely tested as complex genetic influences on disease development are discovered, but their precise impact on our life cycles will be difficult to measure. There is little doubt, too, that imaging, without the use of invasive procedures, will continue its remarkable evolution, so that early detection of vascular, neoplastic and degenerative diseases can be achieved by direct visualisation rather than by the detection of proxy biological markers – think of colon cancer and faecal occult bloods, coronary heart disease and cholesterol, prostate cancer and prostate specific antigen.

Much of this information will be made available to patients by private organisations that may not be well connected to health services and may not be able to provide adequate interpretation and follow-up of potentially alarming findings.

The use of information communications technology has the potential to change radically the relationships between doctors and patients, at home and in the surgery, by the use of text and picture messaging, of remote biosensors and even remote testing for monitoring chronic disease – a potentially chilling alternative to the warm support provided in the practice's chronic disease management clinics.

And there will, of course, be more unpredictable changes. But at the centre there will always be a patient and a clinician, whose tasks will continue to include coordinating care, providing advice, support and explanation, protecting from harm and encouraging well-being. Roles, responsibilities and medical terminology may all change, but this person looks to me very much like a general practitioner.

Chapter 2 A day in the life of a general practitioner

Richard Savage and Suzanne Savage

Introduction

One of the most attractive features of being a general practitioner (GP) is the variety and flexibility it can bring to a working life, both from day to day and throughout a career. Both authors have lived and worked in London for more than 30 years and have been fortunate to combine family life with fulfilling and varied careers. General practice has allowed us to work full or part-time (Chapters 9 and 11) and combine or change work patterns with time for teaching, research, politics, journalism and sabbatical leave, to name but a few. Unwittingly, we have pursued 'portfolio careers' long before this title was invented.

The majority of GPs still work 'full-time', which usually means eight or more sessions a week. Traditionally, doctors would be partners in their practices sharing the risks and rewards of running a business. Today many doctors choose to take up salaried options and prefer the increased flexibility and freedom from administration and other responsibilities. Others choose to do less clinical work and spend more time managing and developing the practice. Typically 13–20 patients are seen in each surgery (although workload can vary widely). In addition, more consultations are now conducted over the telephone to give advice and discuss results of investigations or patient concerns. Visits are provided for housebound patients and those too ill to come to the surgery.

In most practices the staff will meet at regular intervals to discuss practice policy, to share learning over difficult cases or to learn from critical incidents or other difficulties experienced. The successful working of the whole team from receptionists to nurses and doctors is vital for effective

Choosing General Practice: Your Career Guide. Edited by Anne Hastie and Anne Stephenson. © 2008 Blackwell Publishing, ISBN: 978-1-4501-7070-3.

general practice. Success is not just about the one-to-one relationship with our patients but also the delivery of health education, screening and public health policies. Following guidelines when appropriate, applying protocols and recording data contribute to the provision of 'evidence' to achieve targets set annually by the government in its Quality and Outcome Framework programme, which provides a proportion of our income. The rest of our income mainly comes from the number of patients registered with our practice. Other income can be generated from appointments held outside the practice.

GPs have to be able to run general practice as an efficient business, as well as being competent, up-to-date clinicians. Most GPs employ a practice manager who can be the lynchpin of the business and employment side of the practice and who oversees the running of the practice team.

First and foremost the GP must be a generalist who has highly developed communication skills and an overriding interest in the individual patient and his or her problems. Disease can present at an early, undifferentiated stage and all diseases are seen by the GP. This can be exciting but also challenging. The GP therefore has to be able to cope with uncertainty and be able to hear and understand the patient's story, however painful.[1] Consultations tend to be brief but intense and sometimes may not have obvious clinical content. This is where the training for the speciality of general practice appropriately focuses (Chapter 6).

The following is an abridged, consecutive commentary on the surgery of one of the authors. It may not be typical of a country GP's surgery but the rural GP will also have a similar variety of persons and situations.

Box 2.1 Monday morning, somewhere in London: lives in the day of a GP

Alarm wakes me at 7.25 a.m. I am out of the house by 7.40 a.m. and cycle to work, arriving at 7.55 a.m. Usual banter with staff before the routine of turning on the computer and logging into our appointment system, our GP notes system, Choose & Book, GP Note Book and other sundry programmes that support me while I am working. This process takes about 7 min. Collect 30 or so letters that have accumulated since Friday lunchtime, I read them and decide on which information needs to be added to the computer, which information needs further action and which information needs filing. Check the computer for any pathology results that have been downloaded over the weekend, make decisions about abnormal results and add results to patients' notes. Check and sign 25 repeat prescriptions, reviewing and re-authorising medication where necessary. Get myself a quick cup of coffee before seeing the first patient at 8.30 a.m. Multi-tasking rules OK!

G is upset because her daughter who lives in Italy has been diagnosed with breast cancer. She went out to stay with her and contrasts my consulting room and style with that of the Italian breast specialist who held his consultation in a sumptuously designed living room, greeted her daughter with three kisses European style and behaved as if she was a family member.

My next patient had several symptoms that did not seem to come together. She was widowed and lonely and finding the stress of living on her own difficult to manage. We talked and explored possibilities of how she might start to reconstruct her life.

The next patient spoke no English but by a series of gestures and other non-verbal communication I guessed that he was complaining of some sort of bowel problem. This is not the sort of consultation that the Royal College of General Practitioners examiners would score very highly but at least it might break their monotony and give them something to chuckle at.

An African woman attended who had opacities in both eyes. At the back of her mind was the threat of losing her eyesight and how she might manage if this were to happen. Fortunately her condition did not threaten blindness and I hoped that my reassurance starting from her fears and anxieties might be effective, but time will tell.

The Italian consulting room scenario came into mind again as I had to carry out a speculum examination (having first offered my patient a chaperone which she politely declined). Having used re-sterilisable metal specula for 30 years, Health & Safety have decreed that we can only use disposable ones. These require considerably larger amounts of lubricant, are stiff and not as easy to use and my cynical side resents the bureaucracy that has made this examination less easy to carry out.

Another loner. This time a man in his early fifties who has had his second cerebro-vascular accident which has left him still able to look after himself but with fairly considerable speech impediment and loss of use of his right arm so that he is not able to work. I gave him the results of his blood tests. Raised liver enzymes, five times the upper limit of normal, prompted the inevitable question about whether he was drinking. He smiled wistfully and said that he was averaging two bottles of wine a day. I wondered if I, in his position, might not do exactly the same thing. I dutifully ran through the risk factors and drinking advice which NICE and other learned committees would nod approvingly at whilst at the same time trying to be sympathetic and gaining understanding of this man's extremely difficult position. It is at a time like this that I am grateful for continuity of care because I have known this patient for many years and he has grown to trust and may be even like me a little, so that we are able to be frank with each other about our hopes and expectations. I am left with a feeling of admiration for a man with a severe handicap who is still independent and who might consider modifying his behaviour or who may continue to drink heavily but agreed to give me a progress report in a month or two.

D was next. She is a dis-inhibited obese schizophrenic in her mid-forties with very poorly controlled diabetes, hypertension and is every practice's nightmare when it comes to hitting performance targets in these areas. Although not intentionally disruptive, her dis-inhibited behaviour causes a considerable amount of tension and stress for staff and other patients whenever she attends the surgery. She uses the surgery as an important social centre in her life and values the relationship she has with our staff and doctors. Life has become much more difficult for her since her mother died and although they did not live together her mother was a moderating influence on her more bizarre behaviours and was a source of social contact for her. No amount of caseworker input, community psychiatric nurses, occupational therapy or courses can fill up all the minutes in D's day and so she inevitably finds her way to the surgery almost daily as well as Accident & Emergency about five times a month (cost £120/visit). D is an ideal project for the newly appointed Community Matron!

I then received a telephone call from our primary care trust (PCT) requesting that we organise an urgent meeting with them to discuss 'demand management' (management-speak for knocking 20% of our prescribing budget).

Whilst trying to retrieve the next patient's records my computer crashed and I had to spend 5 minutes rebooting it. We requested a computer system upgrade 8 months ago (the PCT now owns all GP IT equipment) but a £21 million reduction in the PCT's budget and a stolen shipment of computers destined for general practice will mean no new IT equipment for us this year.

My next patient was an old friend who I have known for a very long time. He was an alcoholic 25 years ago. It was very difficult to get him to accept what moderate drinking might be as he previously worked as a waiter in one of the large London hotels and used to recount the numbers of empty bottles that he collected from the suite where Liz Taylor and Richard Burton were staying. His controlled drinking allows him to work full-time and he is about to receive an award from the Council for innovative youth work.

My surgery was then interrupted by an epileptic with severe personality disorder, who barged into my consulting room demanding repeat medication, followed by a flustered receptionist. I tried to pacify both and provided him with the prescription that he was wanting. He in his turn was gracious enough to apologise to the reception staff on his way out (phew – otherwise I might have been asked to remove him from our list because we always support our staff when they are harassed or abused by patients). While all this was going on I collected several telephone numbers of patients to phone back between consultations.

I collect my first home visit request of the day to a woman with a 'pain in the neck'.

I then receive a telephone call from a surgical registrar at King's who has just decided that he wants to change his career and train for general practice before the mandatory 3-year run-through GP specialty training programme starts in August 2007. I give him career advice and point him in the direction of the London GP Deanery to apply to a local scheme.

A young woman arrives who is very tearful and depressed. She has so many terrible things going on in her life that it is hard to know where to start. We agree that medication is not the answer and I refer her to our counsellor who will be able to explore her tragic circumstances in a less hurried way.

I then see an ex-addict who has been clean for several years to treat his allergic conjunctivitis and tinea pedis (athlete's foot).

My next patient arrives with acute painful swelling of his great toe joint. I diagnose gout which is easy to treat.

Then on the emergency list I see a 19-year-old with severe chest pain who had called the ambulance to take him to casualty twice over the weekend. ECG and cardiovascular assessment were normal on both occasions and I ascribed his chest discomfort to his first use of cocaine 3 days previously. He came with his girlfriend and the various options should cocaine become a major problem for him were discussed.

I then saw a 6-year-old girl with a urinary tract infection (subsequently confirmed as E. Coli on the specimen I sent to the laboratory for culture).

Next there was a call from a 92-year-old man with a long-term indwelling urinary catheter who had a recurrence of his antibiotic resistant bladder infection that would require intravenous antibiotic treatment and an admission to hospital.

A 70-year-old attended with left-sided abdominal pain requiring examination and further blood tests.

Then it was time to be off to do my visits and on the way out of the surgery I nearly tripped over a metre square box of condoms that had just arrived from the PCT. Normally this would have cheered me up enormously as we have been trying for years to improve condom usage in our part of London, but it does seem ironic that suddenly there is an oversupply of condoms when we are being asked to cut back on prescribing and hospital referral.

The home visit was to a house that I could not hope to afford as house prices in this part of London have skyrocketed. It was inhabited by a woman and her 10 children and two grandchildren. There was no carpet on the stairs and a cat napped quietly in the darkest corner trying to stay cool in this heat wave. Her neck pain is due to cervical osteoarthritis and is treated accordingly.

On returning to the surgery a partner brings to my attention a patient that we have both seen who was taking four times the recommended dose of digoxin and was starting to feel very unwell. We agreed that we should carry out a critical incident analysis of this potentially serious mistake and this was scheduled for the next practice meeting when we will have gathered more information.

By now it is lunchtime and I grab a sandwich while having some time to myself to go over the events of the morning in case I have forgotten to do something or I have an idea about how to do something better. I then attend our practice meeting which is held fortnightly for an hour and a half and tends to make the day more stressful than usual. There is a lot to discuss, clinical and patient care issues as well as practice organisation and staff management decisions.

The afternoon surgery starts at 3.30 p.m. These appointments are made on the same day so patients attend with acute but usually self-limiting illness. The challenge is to explain and treat while sometimes predicting when health will return. It is important to identify those who are more seriously unwell and require further investigation or referral. I am usually finished by 6.30 p.m. I am tired, but amazed as usual by the variety and conditions of people that I have seen. I thank the staff for their help; we chat and wind down together before I cycle home.

Qualities needed to be a GP

Consider these questions:
• How does this account make you feel?
• Do you think you will be interested and challenged by the kind of situations described?
• What do you think the role of the GP should have been?

- Do you think that doctors should act as clinicians only?
- Would you like to learn the skills needed to manage effectively, both from your point of view as the doctor and that of the patient?
- How should we as GPs respond to society's need for us as an easily accessible and free service?

Potential GPs need to answer these questions for themselves. There is a well-known saying in general practice that 'GPs get the patients they deserve' and certainly if the doctor described above is receptive to hearing the stories of those patients, he or she will attract those who need or want to tell their stories. Another doctor in the same practice might not see any drug addicts by personal choice having gained the agreement by the practice. However, the reality of general practice is that as well as needing skills to be able to diagnose disease from early presentation of indistinct symptoms, we have to also respond to what the patients bring to us.

Roy Porter in his Introduction to the Cambridge History of Medicine[2] outlined the great paradox of twentieth century medicine, 'better health and longer life have been accompanied by even greater medical anxieties'. The GP sees patients who are victims of these anxieties.

Helman[3] described the emergence of five triads that can influence what goes on in the general practitioner's consultation.

1 The 'doctor–patient–manager' implies doctors have obligations to be more efficient and accountable. While these skills are needed to effectively see and treat patients as well as running a business it also currently implies loss of independence as the government takes more control of the NHS.

2 The 'doctor–patient–lawyer' highlights an outcome of the impact of the 'complaint culture' that describes growing mutual suspicion between doctor and patient, the increasingly unrealistic expectations about medical outcomes and increasing anxiety about health and illness as described by Roy Porter.[2]

3 The 'doctor–patient–statistician' describes the influence of 'performance targets' in screening, prescribing, immunisation and referral. The needs of the population can be placed before those of an individual. Committee generated guidelines are seen as 'best practice' or used as 'targets' but there can be a tension between the 'perceived wisdom' of others and the negotiated requirements of an individual patient.[4]

4 The 'doctor–patient–journalist' has benefited patients as they have become better informed from the popular press television and the internet. However, patient expectations can be raised unrealistically leading to dissatisfaction when they are not met. Also more information about risks and unwanted outcomes heighten anxiety. Ill patients may find themselves unable to cope with all this information but unhappy when

the GP cannot meet their expectations. This suggests a further triad of the 'doctor–patient–fear' with patients fearful of information presented in a sensational way to sell copy and doctors fearful of making mistakes with the subsequent threat of litigation.

5 The 'doctor–patient–computer' has transformed general practice from its previous minimal use of technology. Information technology is an indispensable third party to the consultation. It is the talisman of the new health care approach but risks reinforcing the mechanical non-human notion of self[5] and steer the consultation away from the inevitable uncertainty of individual treatment and outcomes. It may also ignore the stress of dealing with emotions and feelings. Data entry can cast the patient as an irrelevant irritation in the struggle to meet the computer's demands.

To Helman's triads we add the role of 'doctor–patient–gatekeeper', the lynchpin in the efficient use of the NHS where GPs were able to refer patients to expensive secondary care when they thought necessary. This system has been criticised for not being open or explicit and for the NHS providing different levels of care for the same conditions. PCTs are currently attempting to set limits to prescribing and referrals and therefore risk turning the judgement about referral into a rationing decision. Attempts to provide a more evenly distributed supply of services may mean that striving for excellence is replaced by minimal standards of patient care. Politicians and health service managers are increasingly influencing decisions about availability and levels of care so clinicians are having this role wrested from them.

We also fulfil the role of 'doctor–patient–advocate'. We might lobby for patients to be seen sooner, be reinstated onto waiting lists and occasionally request funding for services that have been withdrawn from NHS patients. We may advise on issues relating to the workplace, employer relations and access to community-based and other services such as legal advice. We are both fortunate to have a welfare rights worker in our practices so we can delegate financial problems. Housing and homelessness is a major problem for some of our patients and while medical conditions are only a small part of assessing housing priority, directing our patients to discuss their problems with their local MP occasionally produces results.

Summary

From the above it is clear that a career in general practice is not ideal for every doctor. It asks a great deal of the individual.
- There is a need for an inquisitiveness and interest in other people.
- Skills are required to work effectively within a team, sometimes leading but sometimes following and supporting or being supported.

- A reliable and effective support network outside of work is important to cope with the professional and emotional stresses of general practice.
- Being able to adapt and change, have flexibility to alter working patterns and energy and diplomacy to ensure the practice adapts to new challenges.
- Bravery is needed to be able to cope with uncertainty concerning diagnosis and management at the early undifferentiated stage of an illness. You need to take 'the main chance'.
- Stamina is needed to be able to consult with many patients over the course of a day whilst recording medical data effectively.
- Being able to weigh up 'evidence' and keep up to date so that you are learning all the time to become a better clinician is a challenge all GPs need to aspire to.
- Having the humility to admit mistakes and to learn from them is vital.
- Learning about ourselves from our patients as their beliefs challenge our own in intimate areas such as relationships, sexuality and cross cultural issues can be personally threatening and challenging.
- Those of us who tend to be perfectionists may struggle with the difficult concept of 'the good enough doctor' rather than the 'perfect doctor'.

For all its many challenges general practice offers so much to those who aspire to work at the 'front line' or 'coalface' of medicine. It is a unique privilege to be able to sit down beside a patient and listen to their story with unconditional positive regard. The GP's knowledge, humanity, empathy and emotional involvement combine to provide a 'good enough' consultation.

References

1 Heath I (1995) *The Mystery of General Practice*. London: Nuffield Provincial Hospitals Trust.
2 Porter R (ed.) (1996) *The Cambridge Illustrated History of Medicine*. Cambridge: Cambridge University Press.
3 Helman C (2002) The culture of general practice. *British Journal of General Practice* **52**: 619–620.
4 Misselbrook D (2002) *Thinking About Patients*. London: Petroc Press.
5 Turkle S (1984) *The Second Self: Computers and the Human Spirit*. London: Granada.

Chapter 3 **Applying for medical school**

John Rees

Introduction

If you are reading this book then it is likely that you have decided that medicine is the course you are looking for. However, this is an important decision to consider carefully. Medical courses are 5 or 6 years long and are aimed at a vocational training rather than a general degree useful in other fields. The training continues as a postgraduate. Compared to many university degree programmes undergraduate medical programmes are relatively intensive. They are also expensive because of their length and the limited ability to work part-time with the commitments to teaching sessions in different sites. So it is important to explore the area thoroughly first and then decide that medicine is really the right choice for you.

Making the decision to apply

Exploration of the area should begin ideally before making A level choices since the wrong choice may restrict the range of medical schools to which you can apply. The best way to explore at this stage is to talk to current medical students and to recently qualified doctors. Relatives or parents' friends who qualified 20–30 years ago may give you useful information but their knowledge of present undergraduate courses may not be as up to date as you need. They are likely to have memories of working very long hours as junior doctors; the situation has changed markedly for current graduates.

Your school or college may well have contacts with previous pupils who have gone to medical school or qualified more recently. Talk to them about the course or their job. You need to get an idea of the life of a medical student, ask them to take you through a typical week at various stages of the programme. Think how you would find the experience, remembering that you are changing

Choosing General Practice: Your Career Guide. Edited by Anne Hastie and Anne Stephenson. © 2008 Blackwell Publishing, ISBN: 978-1-4501-7070-3.

and maturing and your feelings and priorities are likely to develop over the next 5 to 10 years.

You don't really need to decide anything about the field you will go into at this stage. After reading this book you are likely to be interested in general practice and it is quite likely that you will follow this through and make that your career. Many students though, enter medical school convinced they already know that they are destined to be a paediatrician or a surgeon. As they go through the various specialties and see the options they may change their minds. Medical schools will not expect you to come with your life's career planned out. If you have a strong interest in one area that will be respected but all students will go through the whole range of core attachments and see the possibilities of a large range of available careers.

Choosing the course

There are a number of different courses in medicine. The traditional route for a United Kingdom (UK) medical student has been to take appropriate A levels and enter directly into an undergraduate programme. These may be basic 5-year programmes where an extra year for an intercalated BSc is optional or may be 6 years including 1 year acquiring a degree in one particular area. However, the range of programmes available has broadened over the last few years.

The next biggest group of applicants will be those who go into medicine after doing another first degree. This may be because the decision to do medicine came later, because of failure to gain entry to medicine on leaving school or because their A levels weren't those compatible with entry at that time. Graduate entry may be into a standard 5-year programme when the intercalated degree would not generally be appropriate or into specific graduate entry programmes, most of which are for 4 years. Entry into current graduate programmes is very competitive but the number of graduate places is increasing and at present these carry the added advantage that NHS bursaries are available from the second rather than the fifth year of the course.

Another way into medicine is to take a preparatory year. A few medical schools do a conversion year for those without appropriate science A levels, where success in that year guarantees entry to the medical course. These are likely to cover key scientific areas such as biology, chemistry, physics and maths. In addition there are a number of stand alone premedical courses. These need to be explored very carefully since not all courses are accepted for entry to all medical schools. Look into this carefully with the college running the premedical course and the prospectus of the medical schools you are considering for your application.

Some medical schools are running widening access programmes for targeted groups such as inner city school children who may have had less academic opportunity at school. These generally run for one extra year with an initial year or spreading the first two years over three years to allow some extra time and tutoring. Your school should know if you are likely to be eligible for such a programme.

Overseas applicants to UK medical schools are treated in the same way as British applicants if they come from a country in the European Union (EU) but medical schools are limited in the number of students they are allowed to take from overseas countries outside the EU. At present the maximum number allowed is 7.5% of their total student number.

All courses lead to exactly the same medical qualification at the end and lead into the same training after qualification. In fact when there are a number of streams within the same medical school many of these come together for the later parts of the course.

Choosing a medical school

At present all medical schools arrange their own undergraduate programme and their assessments although these are subject to regular review by the General Medical Council (GMC) which is responsible for overseeing undergraduate medical education in the UK. At present there is consultation about the possibility of a national qualifying examination or common elements in each medical school's examination. This may bring the curricula in different schools closer together but they will retain their own individuality.

There are around 29 medical schools in the United Kingdom and the Universities and Colleges Admissions Service (UCAS) form allows space for you to choose four. Geography may be an important element in your choice. You may want to be in a particular area of the country, close to or far away from your home. In the United Kingdom there has been more of a tradition than in other countries for students to move away from their home area to go to university although this trend has reduced in the last 10 years.

The type of course may influence you. Although most UK courses have a blend of different approaches to learning, some courses have a strong problem-based learning element, some retain more didactic teaching; some have more intensive early clinical contact while others have a more traditional divide after the first two or three years. Some schools continue to have active medical student involvement in dissection as part of their anatomy teaching, others rely on prosection of cadavers by experts for students to see while others have gone away from cadavers and teach their anatomy from interactive computer programmes.

In order to find out about a particular course you should look at the medical school website and investigate their prospectus which will often be available online. This may help to give you a feel of the ethos of their course. If you know people who are studying there or have studied there recently, then talk to them about the way the course works. You may want to explore the extent to which medical students interact with students on other courses in accommodation or social activities.

If you are serious about a particular place then you should visit the campus. The best way to do this is in one of their open days for prospective students. This will usually involve a tour of the facilities and a chance to quiz some of the current students, remembering that the students you see may have been chosen carefully to take around prospective applicants. Visiting the campus will be helpful in getting a feel of the main medical school site but take the opportunity to ask the students about their community and hospital placements and experiences since most of your time in a medical course is likely to be spent away from the main university site. The visit will also be a chance for you to gain information which may be useful if you come to interview at that school.

Filling in your UCAS form

The UCAS forms are changing to an online application but the important elements will remain the same. Your flexibility is in the way you complete your academic achievements and the personal statement. The academic achievements should be clear and accurate. It is important that you are honest and accurate throughout the form. Find out from your school what they intend to give as your predicted A level grades. There is little point applying to a school with predictions which are below their entry requirement since they are likely to have many other applicants who more than match these criteria.

Most schools will not consider applicants who have only obtained their grades at resit examinations unless there are documented mitigating circumstances to explain the poorer results first time. Such mitigating circumstances will require backup from your school or doctor as appropriate. Other qualifications such as the International Baccalaureate or Scottish Highers are welcomed by medical schools.

The personal statement is an area that many students agonise over but many medical schools gloss over quite quickly because they find that the statements tend to be very similar. Some schools will formally score the personal statement as one of their criteria for calling applicants to interview. In the personal statement you need to get over relevant information about yourself and your views. It should have something about your suitability or motivation to do medicine. Some form readers are, perhaps unfairly, suspicious of applicants whose motivation comes from an experience when they were young or a tragedy or illness in a close relative, because they are looking for a mature and considered decision to embark on a medical career.

Make sure that your personal statement is correct in its grammar, spelling and punctuation. Get someone else to read it carefully before submission. Don't feel that you have to fill up every square centimetre of the form. A concise, clear personal statement covering the important areas will be welcomed.

Medical schools will normally expect to see mention in the personal statement of work experience. Since the form is submitted in October you will probably have completed the work experience but, if not, you should describe your plans for this to happen soon. They will also like to see some evidence of social or community commitment and the ways you spend your time outside academic activity. This may be playing a musical instrument, sport, reading or other interest. This may be an opportunity to show that you are a good contributor to a team effort. They want to see that you are a rounded person, that you don't have to spend every minute working to get your academic grades and that you have interests that you are likely to maintain when you come to medical school. Again you must be honest. If you claim to have Grade 8 flute they might just produce one for you to play, or at least they are likely to explore this interest in an interview.

Work experience

You will need to get some work experience. This is a reasonable expectation since it shows that you have explored the career seriously and know what you are letting yourself in for. Work experience can be difficult to obtain unless there are arrangements through your school or your family and friends. Otherwise you will need to approach local hospitals, hospices and nursing homes and your general practitioner. Do this in good time since the arrangements may take some time to organise. There will be restrictions on what you can observe but it will give you an opportunity to be in the medical environment and to talk to health professionals and to patients. You may be able to get experience by volunteering to help in some way in a residential or nursing home or a surgery. This may not put you directly in the clinical team but you will gain suitable experience by being in the environment and part of the team and will get opportunities to talk to those working there.

Make sure that you reflect on what you saw during the work experience and your reaction to it. This will help develop your thoughts about medicine and provide evidence at interview that you are able to think about your experiences and are able to reflect and learn from them. It is often helpful to take the time to write these things down soon after the work experience and to remember some things that really made an impression such as particular patients or conversations with staff. Talk to all the staff, not just doctors. Medicine is practised in a multidisciplinary environment and you should be able to see how these teams of doctors, nurses, physiotherapists, social workers, porters, etc. all work together for the good of the patient. In an interview it is likely that you will be asked something about team work, your experience of it as a member or observer of a team.

The other good way to find out what studying medicine is really like and what your response may be is to sign up for one of the programmes such as Medlink which is designed for students exploring medicine as an option. It will give you an opportunity to meet and talk to other potential medical students.

Aptitude testing

Aptitude testing has been used by selected medical schools for some years and in 2006 a new test the UK Clinical Aptitude Test (UKCAT) was introduced for the majority of schools. Some schools have retained their other tests, the BioMedical Admissions Test (BMAT) test which includes an element of General Certificate of Secondary Education (GCSE) science to test knowledge retention and, for graduate entry courses, the Medical Schools Admissions Test (MSAT) and the Graduate Australia Medical School Admissions Test (GAMSAT), the latter is used widely in Australian medical schools. The MSAT consists of sections on critical reasoning, interpersonal understanding and written communication but no factual scientific knowledge and can be used by schools interested in the reasoning ability of arts or science students and GAMSAT also includes a significant science knowledge element.

The UKCAT is an onscreen test that lasts around two hours. Information about the test and registration can be found at: http://www.ukcat.ac.uk/home/. Registration for the test starts in early June and the test must be completed by late September. In the UK it is claimed that every applicant should be within 40 miles of a test centre and 80% will be within 20 miles. There are many testing centres throughout the world, although there are exemptions for candidates from a number of countries such as China. At present the test costs £60 for EU applicants and £95 outside the EU. There is a bursary scheme through which the test fee can be waived for those who receive certain state educational benefits in EU countries. There are four testing areas, each containing around 40 questions:

- *Verbal reasoning:* ability to think logically about written information and arrive at a reasoned conclusion
- *Quantitative reasoning:* ability to solve numerical problems
- *Abstract reasoning:* ability to infer relationships from information by convergent and divergent thinking
- *Decision analysis:* ability to deal with various forms of information, to infer relationships, to make informed judgements, and to decide on an appropriate response in situations of complexity and ambiguity.

The website contains some examples of each section. These can be tried and the answers and explanations are also provided. Schools are free to use the results of the UKCAT as they like and this is likely to change over the next few years. Initially most schools may well look at the results alongside their current arrangements for assessment of academic ability, references and personal statements from UCAS forms. If they become more confident in the UKCAT results then those schools with large numbers of applicants may well use a cut-off score from the test to just look more closely at applicants who score above this threshold.

It is said that the results of the aptitude tests with no knowledge content such as the UKCAT and MSAT are not changed by preparation or practice. Those with a knowledge content such as GAMSAT have spawned a large number of commercial courses aimed at improving performance in the test. Although no specific training is likely to be helpful for UKCAT and MSAT it is certainly worth becoming familiar with the format of these aptitude tests, so that they are not a surprise on the day, and preparing with some practice on similar tests in examination-type conditions. Look carefully at the websites and the example questions to limit any surprises on the day of the test.

The interview

Most UK medical schools interview selected prospective candidates and these interviews take a variety of forms. Most of them have an element of structure in their format. Reliability in interviewing is improved by a structured or semi-structured format. They are likely to cover current academic progress, motivation for the choice of medicine, work experience, social or community involvement, evidence of teamwork and outside interests.

Some details of the form of the interview should be available beforehand such as the place, length and number on the panel. Some schools include current students in their interview panel. It is probably sensible to dress in the way you might expect a clinical medical student to dress, cleanly, tidily and relatively conservatively.

Some schools are moving away from simple interviews to assessment by observing interaction or team work or by giving candidates specific tasks and seeing how they adapt to them. Some use a sequence of short tasks or multiple mini interviews. Some schools have combined their admission process into selection centres where a number of schools combine in running selection days. This may help in limiting the amount of time an applicant has to devote to interviews. Each school is then able to use the results from the selection centre as part of their individual process. Once again the format should be available to you before the interview. In addition there are a number of unofficial websites where applicants share their experiences. These have no sanction from the medical schools but may provide some useful informal and uncensored information for applicants.

Some medical schools provide an ethical issue for discussion just before the interview. If this is the case then it is not meant to have a right or wrong answer but to be a vehicle to see how you go about looking at both sides of an argument. Often this will involve seeing things from the doctor's and the patient's or society's viewpoint. It is likely to be helpful for this and other parts of the interview if you keep up to date with medical issues appearing in the major newspapers over the weeks or months before your interview. Remember that interviewers will often have your UCAS form in front of them and are likely to want to explore some of the things you have written about on the form. Take the opportunity to read your own personal statement again before you go to the interview.

Often you will be asked at the end of an interview whether you have any questions for the interview panel. Do not think that you have to ask something. Responding that you have read the prospectus, or been to the open day or talked to current students and had your questions answered already is fine. However, if you do have a genuine question not answered elsewhere this is your chance to ask it.

In general, interviews do not explore factual medical information but the panel may well expect you to know something about topics that you have highlighted on your personal statement. This is considered reasonable since you have opened the topic by mentioning it on your form.

Even though you will almost certainly be nervous in the interview, one of the most important elements is to get across your enthusiasm and interest. Your interviewers are likely to be favourably influenced by finding someone who looks as if they would be fun to teach and will be keen to learn. So, without gushing too much you need to give that impression. Be yourself but be suitably animated. If the interviewers struggle to get you to engage in conversation they are unlikely to be favourably impressed by your likely communication skills when you get to meet patients. Most schools have a good number of candidates to choose from, many of whom would succeed very well as medical students. You need to show why you are one of the number they should choose from this group.

Gap years

A minority of school leavers opt to do a gap year before going to university. If you intend to do this you can either apply with your predicted grades before you go away or the following year when you already have your A level results. This probably puts you in a stronger position if your results are good but you may find it easier to apply and get your place sorted before going on your gap year because of potential travel difficulties with interviews. In general, medical schools welcome gap years and accept deferred entry but expect the gap year to have some useful structure. This doesn't necessarily need to be solely in a health field, but should have some experience which usually has a health, social or community dimension lasting for a significant period. They understand that much of the rest of the year will have to be spent raising money for the more constructive element of the year.

Summary

The most important element of application to medical school is to explore medicine as a career. You need to do this to make sure that medicine is really for you and to show that you are serious about the application. Research the medical schools that interest you, their requirements and the processes they use in selecting their students. Medical schools will be impressed that this shows an active enquiring learning style.

Chapter 4 **Undergraduate training**

Helen Graham

Introduction

When you begin a medical degree, you are also starting your career in medicine. You are embarking on an exciting and demanding course that requires systematic study in order to achieve the standards required to graduate and begin the next part of training as a pre-registration doctor (Figure 4.1).

The length of training depends on the programme onto which you have been accepted. The standard programme takes 5 years of full-time study, the accelerated graduate entry programme takes 4 years, students taking a 1-year pre-medical or foundation year will progress to the main medicine programme completing their studies in 6 years, while students on an 'Access' programme (Southampton, King's) will take 6 years to cover the same curriculum as the standard programme. All programmes lead to the award of Bachelor of Medicine and Bachelor of Surgery although the exact letters of the award vary from university to university (MBBS; MBChB, MBBChir). All medical schools offer the option of extending the undergraduate programme by 1 year to study for a science honours degree (BSc Hons, BA at Oxford) known as an intercalated degree. Some medical schools offer an opportunity to combine the standard medical with a PhD programme, an option intended for exceptional students interested in a career in research. Manchester offers a combined degree of Medicine with European studies.

What will I study?

During the medical course you will learn about health, illness and the treatment of disease in patients, populations and society. The course aims for you to become a competent doctor in a modern changing health service. You will acquire the knowledge, skills and attitudes necessary to become a

Choosing General Practice: Your Career Guide. Edited by Anne Hastie and Anne Stephenson. © 2008 Blackwell Publishing, ISBN: 978-1-4501-7070-3.

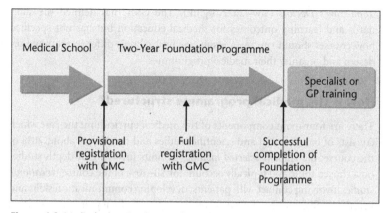

Figure 4.1 Medical education from undergraduate to general postgraduate training.

doctor. You will be expected to take responsibility for your own learning and to think critically, supported by your teachers who will act as guides to support your progress. The medical course is demanding, intellectually, physically and emotionally, and will prepare you for a professional life which involves hard work, a keen interest in people and the ability to apply scientific and clinical principles to the wide range of problems for which patients seek help. Not only will you study the science that underpins the practice of medicine, but also, to become a caring and compassionate doctor, you need to understand patients' social, psychological and emotional needs and how these affect the way they cope with illness and the consequences of their illness.

The study hours required for medicine exceed those of most other under-graduate courses. In the early years, teaching will be based on a university campus and nearby teaching hospitals and general practices, but in later years the clinical course will be located away from the university in hospitals and general practices distributed throughout the region linked to the medical school. This will necessitate a great deal of travelling as well as spending considerable time living away from your university city. Academic terms are longer than standard university terms, up to 32 weeks in the first two years, and up to 48 weeks in years 3, 4 and 5. This restricts the potential to work to supplement your income, and leaves only 4 weeks of annual holiday.

Medical degree programmes in the United Kingdom are broadly similar and are based on a modern curriculum which aims to prepare students to be-come competent doctors working in the National Health Service. All medical schools base their curriculum on recommendations made by the General Medical Council (GMC) for medical education set out in the document

Tomorrow's Doctors (www.gmc.org.uk). The GMC has defined the standards and learning outcomes for medical education but has not specified how courses should run. As a result, medical schools differ in the way they design and organise their medical programmes.

How is the medical programme structured?

There are four main components of the medical curriculum: the *core* which consists of basic clinical and scientific studies and constitutes about 70% of the course; the *student-selected modules* or units involving in-depth studies on a chosen topic and typically account for 20–30% of the course; *vocational studies* involving contact with patients, developing communication skills and practical skills; and the *clinical apprenticeship* in the final year when students learn about being a doctor in hospital and general practice. The practice of medicine demands the highest standards of professional and personal conduct and part of the course will also be concerned with *personal and professional development.*

Most curricula follow a learning spiral with emphasis shifting progressively from medical science to clinical practice as you progress through the course (Figure 4.2). You will start by studying the human basis of medicine and body systems, and linking basic medical sciences with clinical medicine. Following an introduction to medical studies and medical sciences, the course will progress to more detailed teaching on human structure (anatomy), body functioning (physiology) and other essential biomedical sciences including biochemistry, genetics, immunology and the behavioural sciences such as sociology and psychology including ethics and law. Schools have different approaches to teaching anatomy which may involve the

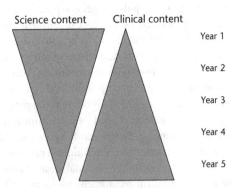

Science content   Clinical content

Year 1

Year 2

Year 3

Year 4

Year 5

Figure 4.2 The vertical integration of subjects in the medical curriculum.

dissection of cadavers, surface anatomy, 3D medical imaging and live dissected models.

Medical schools aim to integrate learning in their programmes but differ in the way they achieve this. Some do so through lectures based on weekly clinical patient cases or scenarios which are supported by seminars, tutorials, laboratory class work and interactive web-based learning. Other schools deliver *systems-based learning* in which lectures and tutorials are grouped and integrated around the different body systems (cardiovascular, respiratory, gastrointestinal, musculoskeletal, skin, nervous, genitourinary, endocrine, reproductive, haematology, immunology and pharmacology) as at Oxford, Sheffield and Nottingham. Other schools such as Manchester, Liverpool, Glasgow and Edinburgh and the newer schools have developed curricula delivered through *problem-based learning* in which a problem-solving approach is applied to a patient's clinical problems. This educational process encourages students to learn through curiosity and seek out information for themselves, working in small groups and using a range of learning resources from the libraries and web-based learning. The advantage of this method is that it helps to lay the foundations for managing students' own future education and career as *life-long learners.*

Medical programmes are structured around years, phases or stages, which may or may not correlate with the years of the programme. This can be very confusing to begin with but allows students on shortened or extended programmes to enter the same phase of the course after 2 years' study as students from a standard course (Figure 4.3). Learning will be shared in parts of the course with mixed professional student groups such as nurses, pharmacists, physiotherapists and dentists and is timetabled as *inter-professional learning.* The purpose of this is to prepare students from different healthcare programmes to work together as teams providing patient care in hospitals, community and general practice.

When will I start to meet patients?

The majority of medical schools offer clinical experience from the start of the course and in a variety of clinical settings, although a few schools delay this until the second year. You can expect to meet patients in hospitals, general practices or in their own homes and you will learn to take a medical history and examine patients. Some schools arrange for a family attachment to a pregnant mother with a new baby (King's) or to an elderly person with a carer (Edinburgh). Early patient contact helps to integrate theory with clinical medicine, and helps to keep you focussed on the reason for studying medicine. During the first year you will meet patients on only a few days but by the third

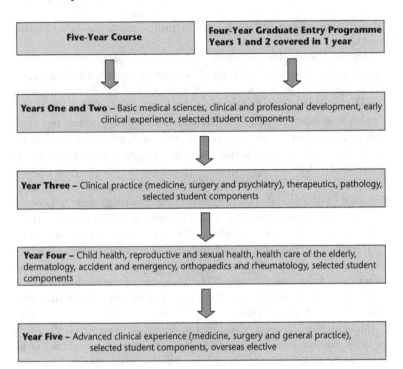

Figure 4.3 Structure of the medical curriculum.

year clinical attachments form the major part of the course. Most schools teach communication and clinical examination early on in the course so that you learn to communicate effectively with people and to behave in a professional role. Many medical schools have a purpose-built clinical skills centre and use actors in teaching communication which helps to develop greater confidence in meeting patients.

What is the clinical course like?

After the second or third year, the course will become more clinically based and you will spend more time in clinical settings, gaining experience on hospital wards, outpatient clinics, general practice, and learning practical clinical skills under supervision. Generally, students start with an introduction to clinical methods and then progress through a series of attachments in surgery, medicine and psychiatry. You will learn in small groups on hospital units called *firms* supervised by a clinical tutor, while in general practice you will be attached in small groups, pairs or one-to-one and under the supervision of a general practice tutor. At this stage you will undertake detailed histories and examination of patients, learn a wide range of clinical skills and have enough clinical knowledge to start diagnosing patients' problems.

In the second clinical year (fourth year of the standard programme) you will have attachments in specialties such as child health and paediatrics, women's health, medicine of old age and degenerative diseases, sexual medicine, accident and emergency medicine, and trauma and orthopaedics. These attachments will be complemented by teaching in clinical sciences with pathology, public health and therapeutics, gaining practical knowledge of drugs and prescribing. The final year usually starts with or includes an *elective* and 6–9 months of a clinical apprenticeship. This will involve shadowing a junior doctor in hospital and a general practitioner in family practice and taking clinical responsibility under supervision in preparation for working as a doctor. Towards the end of the year, you will take the final examination which leads to graduation as a doctor ready to start the Foundation Programme.

Will I have opportunities to choose what I study?

Throughout the medical programme, you will have the opportunity to study subjects of your own choice in depth within an area relevant to medicine which are known as *special study modules* or *student selected components*. You will choose a specialist topic that particularly interests you from a wide range of disciplines with a biomedical, clinical, educational or social component. By studying a subject in depth, you will learn to assess scientific evidence, gain an introduction to research methods or have a taster in a discipline you may wish to consider as a career option. Other study modules are designed to broaden your knowledge or experience, or learn a language useful for an overseas elective. Multi-faculty universities may offer a wide range of subjects drawn from their different schools. For example King's offers an exciting range of modules from specialist subjects in basic medical and clinical sciences in addition to modern languages such as Spanish or Arabic, library projects and modules entitled 'teaching children about health', 'care of the elderly', 'demography of aging', 'drug design and development', 'gene cloning and analysis' and 'sign language'. Arrangements for the choice component of the course vary from school to school with some rotating students into blocks of selected student components while others allocating 1 day each week to them.

The intercalated degree offers further opportunities to spend a year studying a subject in depth. The proportion of students taking this option varies from school to school. All students at Cambridge, Oxford and Imperial take a degree year; other schools offer all students this option, while some other schools restrict this to the more able students. The intercalating degree course is usually taken at the end of the second or third year, although some schools offer flexibility with the timing. At Imperial College, the BSc year counts towards the selected options part of the medical programme. In addition to selected student components, there is an elective which extends from 4–10 weeks and is taken either at the end of the fourth year or during the fifth year. The elective is a period taken away from your university with the purpose of exploring an area of medical practice that excites you, and which you will write up as a project as part of your overall assessment. Most students spend their elective abroad on attachments in hospital or community services experiencing medicine in the developing world, while other students may arrange an attachment in the United Kingdom. The possibilities for electives are endless and may include internships with international organisations such as the WHO or UNESCO.

On graduate entry programmes, students take an accelerated course for the first 1–2 years, covering 2 years' work in one, and then follow the same clinical course as students on the later years of the standard course. At some schools, graduate entry students may be based on a separate campus as at Swansea Clinical School where students later join the Cardiff third year programme and at Derby where students join the Nottingham programme.

How will I be assessed?

Assessment is an important part of the medical programme and demonstrates that you have achieved the standards required for each part of the course. Progress will be assessed in each phase or stage of the course, and will use a mix of factual tests and practical patient-based skills assessments. Progression to the next part of course is dependent on passing. Personal and professional attitudes and behaviour may be assessed at interviews during the clinical attachments. Throughout the course there will be emphasis on learning and assessment of clinical and communication skills and you will be assessed on your competence during the course and in formal clinical examinations. You will have a logbook or electronic learning portfolio (Edinburgh and Newcastle) in which the results of the assessments will be recorded. Distinctions and merits will be awarded for outstanding results in individual units of the programme.

Pastoral care and academic support

Personal development and support at medical school is important. You will be supported by an allocated personal tutor or clinical advisor whom you will meet several times each year to discuss your academic progress, social life and general development. In addition, there will be year coordinators and facilitators for problem-based learning groups, and tutors with special responsibility for students with disabilities such as dyslexia, or other difficulties. The medical school will have staff who will advise you on financial support and the many bursaries and scholarships available to medical students. Some schools have student support arrangements such as peer groups, buddies or 'mums and dads' schemes as at Aberdeen where students are linked with another student in the year ahead for support and advice based on their own experiences.

Student life

Life as a medical student is not all work and no play, and you will make many friends. Most medical schools are part of a multi-faculty university with students' unions and a range of social, sporting and cultural opportunities in university clubs, medical school activities and halls of residence or colleges. Traditionally universities have a protected half-day for social activities, although the first year graduate entry course students will need to study during this time in order to complete their accelerated curriculum. In the later years of the medical course, you may be away from your university base on placements in different parts of the country and so will be unable to participate in the university social life, but you will be learning in small groups and will have personal contact with teaching staff and hospital facilities.

Chapter 5 **Foundation training**

Jan Welch

Introduction

Since 2005 all doctors qualifying in the United Kingdom have to complete a 2-year foundation programme before progressing to further training. The first year encompasses what was previously called the pre-registration house officer year, and leads to full registration with the General Medical Council (GMC). The second year provides further training in the management of acutely ill patients as well as in the generic skills necessary for effective medical practice, such as communication and time management.

In the past early medical training was experiential and somewhat ad hoc. The foundation programme is distinguished by having a clearly defined curriculum and objectively assessed competencies. Trainees are expected to take responsibility for their own learning, both during foundation training and in preparation for continuing professional development. They should engage fully with available educational opportunities as well as ensuring that they carry out the necessary assessments and use their learning portfolios effectively.

The foundation programme formed the first part of the complete restructuring of medical training termed 'Modernising Medical Careers' (MMC).[1] Further information about MMC is available on the website www.mmc.mhs.uk.

What is foundation training?

Foundation training is a 2-year programme bridging the undergraduate years and further training leading to careers in general practice or in a specialty such as medicine or surgery. The 2 years may be based in two separate geographical locations, although each year is usually centred in one hospital. The 2-year

---

Choosing General Practice: Your Career Guide. Edited by Anne Hastie and Anne Stephenson. © 2008 Blackwell Publishing, ISBN: 978-1-4501-7070-3.

programme is educationally balanced to provide a variety of placements rather than focusing on a specialty area.

Nomenclature

Instead of being called pre-registration house officers (PRHOs), the official term for a first year foundation (F1) trainee is foundation house officer 1; in the second year (F2) this becomes foundation house officer 2. The term 'foundation doctor' is preferred for name badges.

The F1 year

The first year supersedes the pre-registration house officer year but still leads to full registration with the GMC. The programme is based on the GMC publication *The New Doctor* and takes account of the GMC's *Good Medical Practice*.

The F1 year must provide sufficient experience in medicine and surgery to meet the GMC outcomes and foundation comprehencies, but may also include experience in other areas such as paediatrics or intensive care. Foundation doctors usually rotate between specialty areas every 3 or 4 months. By the end of the F1 year it is expected that a trainee will be able to manage common clinical situations successfully.

The F2 year

As well as consolidating skills learnt in the F1 year, the F2 trainee is expected to become increasingly proficient in managing acute illness and in appreciating broader aspects of patient care and safety.

The F2 year usually comprises three placements, each of 4 months. One of the 4-month periods is generally spent in emergency medicine or another area able to provide training in acute assessment and care. About 55% of F2 programmes include a general practice placement. Other possible placements enable trainees to experience specialties not usually included within F1 programmes, such as anaesthetics, genitourinary medicine, obstetrics and gynaecology, pathology, psychiatry and public health.

'Tasters' of 1–2 weeks are available as an option during the F2 year. They enable trainees to gain an insight into areas they may be considering for their future careers, but have not had previous opportunities to experience, for example diagnostic specialties such as radiology or pathology.

Training abroad for the F2 year is feasible but needs to be planned well in advance, and prospectively agreed to by the Foundation School

Director and Postgraduate Dean. The placement must be able to deliver training in the required F2 competencies, and provide educational supervision and completion of the assessment tools and learning portfolio.

Responsibility for accrediting the F2 year lies with the Postgraduate Medical Education and Training Board (PMETB).

Academic foundation programmes

Academic foundation programmes have been developed to enable trainees considering an academic career to explore this in more depth. There are various models, with both 1- and 2-year programmes available. Commonly a 4-month period in the F2 year is based in a university laboratory or other academic area, with academic mentorship and training provided during the remaining 8 months of clinical F2 training.

Obtaining a foundation programme

Recruitment to foundation programmes is an online national process. This is now run by the UK Foundation Programme Office (UKFPO) (www.foundationprogramme.nhs.uk).

Foundation training programmes generally start at the beginning of August each year. Applicants, usually final year medical students, apply in the autumn before they expect to start by completing the online application form. In addition, their medical schools have to provide some information including the students' academic rankings.

Applicants have to rank all foundation schools in order of preference. Their application forms are then scored by the applicant's first choice foundation school, by a panel including a clinician, according to nationally agreed scoring guidelines. Application forms are audited and checks made for plagiarism.

Applicants to foundation schools are allocated on the basis of their scores and academic rankings. Foundation schools are then responsible for allocating F1 and F2 training programmes to the trainees within their schools. The employing trusts will carry out checks on references and other pre-employment checks such as occupational health assessment.

The foundation curriculum[2]

The programme is based on a 'spiral curriculum', in that expertise develops from revisiting previous experiences within a variety of settings and advancing complexities. Both training and assessment are workplace based, with experiential learning opportunities presented by ward rounds, clinics, and theatre and investigation sessions. These are supplemented by small group sessions, one-to-one teaching, external courses such as life support or simulator training, and personal study including electronic learning packages, which are becoming increasingly available and useful.

As well as developing clinical skills, the foundation doctor is expected to demonstrate competency in other areas including clinical governance, team working and establishing successful professional relationships with patients. The core competencies for the foundation years are based on the principles outlined by the GMC in its publication *Good Medical Practice*.[3]

These are:

- Good clinical care
- Maintaining good medical practice
- Partnership with patients
- Working with colleagues and in teams
- Assuring and improving the quality of teams
- Teaching and training
- Probity
- Health.

The *Curriculum for the Foundation Years in Postgraduate Education and Training* is published on the MMC website (www.mmc.nhs.uk) with a second edition due to be produced in 2007.

Career management

Career planning is a crucial part of Modernising Medical Careers.[4] Resources have been provided for foundation schools to provide support for doctors in planning and managing their careers. Such support is now available within medical schools and hospitals as well as online via foundation school and postgraduate deanery websites.

In the past many young doctors spent years in senior house officer posts awaiting entry to the specialist registrar grade. Part of Modernising Medical Careers is to enable more streamlined training for those appointed to post foundation training: the 'run-through grade'. Not all trainees, however, will be able to gain entry to their first choice of career, especially in a popular geographical area, and so may need to make alternative plans.

How is foundation training organised?

The educational infrastructure for foundation training is described in the *Operational Framework for Foundation Training* published on the website www.foundationprogramme.nhs.uk.

Foundation schools

Foundation training is overseen by foundation schools, which are developed in collaboration between medical schools and postgraduate deaneries. A foundation school will have a director, supported by a manager and other administrative support, and links with a career advisor or manager. There may be several foundation schools within one deanery. A foundation school may contain several hundred F1 and F2 trainees, in a number of different NHS trusts spanning a wide geographical area.

Foundation schools are responsible for the operational aspects of delivering foundation programmes. These include participation in national processes for recruitment of trainees to the school, allocation of foundation programmes to trainees within the school, overseeing the delivery of training programmes, communicating with trainers and trainees and managing aspects such as trainees who fail to progress or who need alterations to their training programmes for reasons such as maternity leave or illness. Although deaneries are responsible for overseeing the local quality assurance of foundation training, operationally this is being increasingly delegated to the foundation schools.

Foundation training programmes

Foundation training programmes are the managerial unit responsible for local delivery of foundation training within foundation schools. Each contains about 20–40 F1/F2 1-year programmes and is led by a foundation training programme director (FTPD), who is usually a consultant with expertise in medical education. In some cases a clinical tutor/director of medical education may also act as a FTPD.

NHS trusts

Foundation doctors are employed by NHS trusts, not foundation schools. The trusts therefore have responsibility for hours of work and pay banding arrangements as well as ensuring that the local environment meets educational standards, and that local trainers have the time and training to work effectively.

Educational and clinical supervisors

Every foundation trainee has a named educational supervisor. This individual is a senior clinician with expertise in medical education who is responsible for providing regular formative appraisal, supporting the trainees with their learning portfolio and engagement with assessment processes, and ensuring that their training needs are met. The educational supervisor may supervise trainees throughout their F1 or F2 year, or just for the duration of one of the constituent placements, for example in general practice.

Day-to-day supervision of a foundation doctor's clinical and professional practice within a placement is provided by their clinical supervisor, who is usually a consultant in that specialty or a general practitioner. In addition, the clinical supervisor will support the assessment process and ensure that appropriate clinical opportunities are available.

Feedback and assessment

Assessment of foundation doctors is based on evaluation of their competence in workplace settings such as a ward or surgery. It is developmental in that feedback is provided by a supervisor in order to guide further development of the trainee's practice. It is an open and transparent process which should be led by the trainee, although encouragement may be required. Assessment will also determine whether foundation doctors have reached the necessary standard to progress to the next stage.

The learning portfolio

The portfolio is based on the foundation curriculum.[5] The aim is to encourage trainees to develop good practice and reflective learning as well as to assist them in structuring a record of their experience, training, assessments of competence and career management information.

Although the learning portfolio is available in paper form, electronic versions are becoming increasingly used. The portfolio should be available for review at meetings between the foundation doctor and his or her educational supervisor, and should include outcomes of appraisal discussions.

Assessment tools

The tools are described fully in the curriculum and sample forms are available in the learning portfolio. Electronic versions are increasingly being adopted. The first three of these assessment tools capture direct observation of doctor–patient interactions. Developmental feedback is a key part of each exercise.

Mini Clinical Evaluation Exercise (mini-CEX)

This is the evaluation of an observed clinical encounter selected by the trainee, for example the assessment of a patient with a neurological problem at the end of a ward round. The observer, who may be a GP, consultant or experienced specialist or specialty training registrar (SpR/StR), then provides feedback to support further development of the trainee's practice.

Direct Observation of Procedural Skills (DOPS)

DOPS is the observation of a practical procedure, such as urethral catheterisation, selected by the trainee. The observer may be a GP, consultant, experienced SpR/StR or a suitable nurse or allied health professional who has been trained in evaluating the procedure and providing developmental feedback.

Case-based Discussion (CBD)

This is structured discussion of a clinical case to allow exploration of the doctor's reasoning and decision-making, for example using the notes of a patient whom the trainee has seen in outpatients. The discussion should include evaluation of medical record keeping, clinical assessment, investigation and referrals, follow-up and professionalism.

Multi-source Feedback (MSF)

In multi-source feedback 10–12 colleagues selected by the trainee, such as GP principals, consultants, SpRs and experienced nurses are invited to provide feedback on the foundation doctor's attitudes and behaviour using the mini-PAT (peer assessment tool) or TAB (team assessment of behaviour) forms. The results are collated and discussed with the trainee at an appraisal meeting with the educational supervisor.

Summary

The introduction of a 2-year foundation programme with regular assessments should ensure that doctors entering specialty training have acquired appropriate skills.[6] In addition, doctors who will be working in non-training grades should also have obtained the foundation competencies, ensuring the quality of patient care. Doctors should have a better understanding of the career opportunities available, which may alter their original career choice.

References

1 Modernising Medical Careers (2005) *Operational Framework for Foundation Training*. London: The Stationery Office.
2 Modernising Medical Careers (2005) *Curriculum for the Foundation Years in Postgraduate Education and Training*. London: The Stationery Office.
3 General Medical Council (2006) *Good Medical Practice: Guidance for Doctors*. London: General Medical Council.

4 Modernising Medical Careers Working Group for Career Management (2005) *Career Management: An Approach for Medical Schools, Deaneries, Royal Colleges and Trusts.* London: The Stationery Office.

5 Modernising Medical Careers (2005) *Foundation Learning Portfolio.* www.mmc.nhs.uk

6 General Medical Council (2005) *The New Doctor: Recommendations on General Clinical Training,* transitional edition. London: General Medical Council.

Chapter 6 **Specialty training for general practice**

Tim Swanwick

Introduction

Under the auspices of the Department of Health's policy of *Modernising Medical Careers* (MMC) postgraduate general practice is undergoing its biggest shake up since the introduction of vocational training in the 1970s. At that time the Royal College of General Practitioners (RCGP) presented strong evidence to the government to support a 5-year training programme, incorporating 2 years based in primary care. The outcome for those lucky enough to find a structured vocational training scheme was a 3-year programme, a compromise with which general practice has lived ever since. Almost invariably two of those years (sometimes longer for those constructing their own programme) were spent in a selection of hospital posts with just 12 months in the destination specialty of general practice. It is perhaps not surprising that general practice registrars found themselves unprepared for independent practice on exiting training and reluctant to take up substantive posts.[1,2] To compensate for the inadequate training time spent in general practice the Department of Health funded a period of post-certification Higher Professional Education (HPE).[3] The scheme ran for just 3 years (2003–2006) but was then withdrawn on the basis that MMC and the new *speciality training programmes* for general practice would adequately prepare GP trainees for the future.

MMC[4] takes its name from one of a series of policy documents that appeared on the back of a report on the future of the SHO grade by the current Chief Medical Officer, Sir Liam Donaldson. *Unfinished Business*[5] took as its starting point the Calman reforms of the 1990s that had successfully modernised the training of specialist registrars. Donaldson highlighted that SHOs had become a 'lost tribe', waiting (sometimes for years) to enter specialist

---

Choosing General Practice: Your Career Guide. Edited by Anne Hastie and Anne Stephenson. © 2008 Blackwell Publishing, ISBN: 978-1-4501-7070-3.

training with very little in the way of structured education or supervision. He proposed two major pieces of reform to deal with this problem: the establishment of a structured 2-year Foundation Programme during which trainees could sample various specialties (including general practice) before deciding on their future career, and the introduction of structured run-through training programmes into which foundation trainees would pass, eventually resulting in the achievement of a Certificate of Completion of Training (CCT) in their chosen specialty. The net effect of the latter being to reduce the waiting time for entry into specialist training programmes, and therefore reduce the time taken (and cost) to train a specialist consultant or general practitioner.

The Foundation Programme went 'live' in 2005 and to a large extent has achieved its aims. Fifty five percent of all foundation trainees in England now benefit from a substantive general practice experience in their second foundation year, with a significant proportion of trainees following suit in the other UK countries. The second phase of MMC, the introduction of run-through specialty training programmes, begins in August 2007. No longer are there SHOs and registrars but run-through trainees or *specialty registrars*. General practice is no longer a special case but just one of 65 specialties governed by a generic set of rules and regulations.

For all specialties MMC has meant the introduction of competency-based curricula and a reform of assessment programmes. The latter has been particularly welcomed in general practice training which for a number of years has been burdened with a dual assessment system: Summative Assessment and the Membership Examination of the Royal College of General Practitioners (MRCGP).

With reform comes new regulation and the Postgraduate Medical Education and Training Board (PMETB) is now firmly established as the 'competent authority' for medical training. PMETB sets standards for training (see Box 6.1) and is responsible for approving curricula, assessment systems, posts and programmes, and quality assures deaneries. Deaneries functioning as virtual postgraduate medical schools, recruit to, commission, manage and deliver training, and are now also responsible for the quality management of their own training programmes.

So what does the new specialty training for general practice have on offer?

Improved recruitment and selection

One of the successes of general practice training in recent years has been the introduction of competency-based selection and assessment centres run by

---

Box 6.1 The PMETB quality domains

Patient safety
Quality assurance, review and evaluation
Equality, diversity and opportunity
Recruitment, selection and appointment
Delivery of curriculum including assessment
Support and development of trainees, trainers and local faculty
Management of education and training
Educational resources and capacity
Outcomes

---

deaneries, a trend that is intended to be followed by other specialities in 2008. Selection for general practice training is now a standardised and rigorous process that adheres to best human resources practice, is valid and reliable and both transparent and fair.

Following an online application, trainees are invited to apply for a shortlisting assessment. This currently (2007) takes the form of two machine-marked examination papers; a 'clinical dilemmas' and a 'situational judgement' paper. Both assess the appropriate application of clinical knowledge in context. *Clinical knowledge and expertise* is just one of the competencies required by the national person specification which is based on the outcome of a triangulated study by Patterson et al.[6] The complete list of attributes assessed at selection includes:

- *Clinical knowledge and expertise:* capacity to apply sound clinical knowledge and awareness of the full investigation of problems
- *Empathy and sensitivity:* capacity and motivation to take in others' perspectives and to treat others with understanding
- *Communication skills:* capacity to adjust behaviour and language as appropriate to the needs of differing situations
- *Conceptual thinking and problem solving:* capacity to think beyond the obvious, with an analytical and flexible mind
- *Coping with pressure:* capacity to recognise one's own limitations and develop appropriate coping mechanisms
- *Organisation and planning:* capacity to organise information/time effectively in a planned manner
- *Managing others and team involvement:* capacity to work effectively in partnership with others

- *Professional integrity:* capacity and motivation to take responsibility for one's own actions and demonstrate respect for all
- *Learning and personal development:* capacity and motivation to learn from experience and constantly update skills/knowledge.

Following success at shortlisting, candidates are invited to an assessment centre where they undertake a number of observed exercises, which aim to test the range of the competencies listed above. These have included a simulated patient encounter, a group discussion and a written exercise in prioritisation. Success at the assessment centre results in allocation to a Unit of Application – usually coterminus with a deanery. Subsequent allocation to a training scheme, and thence to an individual training programme, is coordinated through the deanery and/or the training programme concerned. The superiority of assessment centres over conventional interviews has been shown in other contexts and feedback from candidates from recent general practice recruitment rounds has been uniformly positive.

Structured training for all

From August 2007, apart from a number of shortened programmes associated with transition, new recruits to general practice will embark on a 3-year training programme. This is a new departure for general practice, as in previous years only 30–40% of UK trainees qualified having undertaken a period of structured training. The majority had constructed their own programme from a mixture of ad hoc SHO posts undertaken both in the United Kingdom and abroad. Following a massive re-badging exercise large numbers of SHO posts have been incorporated into run-through GP training. A further development is the creation of a breed of innovative training posts (ITPs), which are based in general practice but with secondments into the hard-to-access outpatient-based subspecialties such as dermatology, rheumatology, ophthalmology and ENT, as well as into community facilities such as hospices and drug and alcohol units.

In view of the wide-ranging requirements of contemporary general practice all specialty training programmes are required to be broad and balanced. The RCGP has published guidance[7] to assist deaneries as they put together appropriate programmes of training. This guidance states that:

> Programmes should be designed to enable the GP trainee to acquire all the competencies necessary to practise safely and competently in UK general practice and thus should contain an appropriate balance between service and education; hospital medicine, general practice

and experience in other community settings. All the placements that make up the programme should be in specialities that can deliver, in combination, the general practice curriculum competencies. GP training in secondary care should be educationally supervised and monitored from general practice. GP directors should bear in mind that secondary care placements may offer the opportunity to acquire certain competencies much more quickly than is possible in general practice.

A number of specific recommendations are made, namely that programmes should:
- Be completed within 7 years
- Include 18 months as a specialty registrar under the supervision of a GP trainer
- End with a period of at least 6 months in general practice
- Include a minimum of 12 months' training in secondary care specialties
- Include placements in at least three secondary care specialties of 3–6 months' duration
- Include more curriculum relevant hospital placements, e.g. more outpatient and less theatre/ward work
- Include innovative training posts (ITP) enabling trainees to gain experience in larger number of smaller specialties, e.g. dermatology, ENT, eyes, rheumatology
- Be managed by GP specialty programme directors and educational supervision throughout the 3 years from general practice
- Have local flexibility within national guidelines
- Be assessed continually through the workplace-based assessment programme of the MRCGP.

Despite all these developments the RCGP's intention that general practice training programmes should include a minimum of 18 months in practice remains problematic. Although at the time of writing it would appear that around 50% of UK trainees will be offered this opportunity regrettably this has been at the cost of reducing training numbers, a fact that has caused some consternation in workforce planning circles and the '18-month split' remains the subject of high level discussion between deaneries, the Strategic Health Authorities and the Department of Health.

Specialty training programmes, formerly known as vocational training schemes, are looked after by specialty programme directors (formerly known as course organisers). The programme director is a deanery employee and has a number of key roles. He or she is responsible, alone or with others, for the delivery of an appropriate educational curriculum for trainees in general practice. This involves planning, facilitating and evaluating the process of learning. It is the programme director who has the overall responsibility for management of the local programme, ensuring that individual training programmes are broad, balanced and able to deliver the requirements of the RCGP Curriculum. Individual programmes must also be sufficient to enable participation in the MRCGP assessment processes. Within this somewhat dry definition is a multiplicity of complex and interwoven roles, and programme directors are at one and the same time, negotiators, troubleshooters, educational managers, teachers and the deliverers of pastoral care to groups of around 30 trainees.

Educational supervision from general practice

The RCGP Curriculum requires that trainees undertaking programmes in general practice receive educational supervision across their 3-year training. This means that on appointment to a training programme a GP specialty registrar will be allocated to someone who will take an overview of their progress and advise on future learning needs as they progress through training.

In practice, educational supervision will be mediated through the RCGP e-portfolio (see below), which requires a structured review meeting to take place between trainee and supervisor every 6 months. Each review meeting will last 1.5–2 hours and a general discussion takes place about curriculum coverage and the supervisor assesses progress in relation to a number of defined professional competency areas. The trainee provides supporting evidence in the form of workplace-based assessments. It should be noted that these regular reviews do not replace formative meetings with clinical supervisors while the trainee is in secondary care placements, nor those with the GP trainer whilst in practice.

In line with all other specialties, at the end of each year of training, the portfolio of the trainee will be reviewed by a deanery panel and at the end of the training programme as a whole the educational supervisor makes a recommendation to the deanery about whether, in their view, the trainee has reached the required standard. The deanery panel then reviews the portfolio and makes a decision about whether training has been satisfactorily completed and if not whether an extension to training should be granted.

Although this is a departure for some training schemes many have already been running similar local systems of educational supervision, usually through the programme directors. These systems will be superseded by the RCGP portfolio and workplace assessment processes. The regular reviews in the e-portfolio therefore build on what is already considered to be best practice. Educational supervision may be delivered in a number of ways depending on local preference. The role may fall to the programme director or be allocated to a designated trainer for the entire 3 years. Alternatively, and this is the more likely pragmatic compromise, the programme director may assume responsibility but delegate the task of educational supervision to a nominated GP trainer whilst the trainee is in a primary care placement. At the time of writing, the system is as yet untried and unpiloted and no doubt preferred models will arise.

A curriculum for general practice training

Specialty training programmes for general practice then, will be targeted at delivering the competencies of the RCGP Curriculum, a document of which the College can be justifiably proud.

The development of the Curriculum was initiated in 2004 and led by Professor Stephen Field with a small team based at the University of Birmingham. Huge numbers of general practitioners from all over the United Kingdom have contributed to the Curriculum, an impressive document that now runs to some several hundred pages. The RCGP Curriculum was also the first of all the specialty curricula to be approved, in 2006, by PMETB. The Curriculum contains 32 individual 'statements' the most important of which is the first: *Being a General Practitioner*, which forms the backbone of the entire document. The competencies embedded in this core statement run through each of the remaining supporting statements providing the contextual backdrop against which *Being a General Practitioner* is placed.

Being a General Practitioner takes as its starting point the European definition of general practice/family medicine as developed by the World Organisation of Family Doctors (Europe) in 2002[8] and subsequently revised by their education network, the European Academy of Teachers in General Practice in 2006. The decision to use this particular framework was taken because of its educational value, international applicability and acceptability across 30 European countries. As a result of a PMETB curriculum requirement this has meant that a cross-referencing exercise has been necessary to map the RCGP Curriculum against the General Medical Council's *Good Medical Practice.*[9]

Being a General Practitioner describes six holistically defined domains of competence together with three essential features. These are summarised in Box 6.2.

A number of supporting curriculum statements (see Box 6.3) accompany *Being a General Practitioner*. Each statement has broadly the same structure and examines the rationale for including that particular area in a curriculum for general practice alongside the current UK health priorities before defining the knowledge-based and the intended learning outcomes couched in terms of the core competency areas. The supporting statements also provide examples

---

Box 6.2 *Being a general practitioner*: the domains of competence and background features

Six domains of core competence
  Primary care management
  Person-centred care
  Specific problem-solving skills
  Comprehensive approach
  Community orientation
  Holistic approach

The essential background features
  Contextual
  Attitudinal
  Scientific

---

of how the subject might be addressed by both trainees and educators and list relevant further reading and resources.

So what is the purpose of such a collection of documents?

The Curriculum is the bedrock of specialty training and not since *The Future General Practitioner,*[10] published back in 1972, has the field of general practice been so clearly demarcated. That indeed is one of the Curriculum's primary roles, to define the field of study for the learner and how it may be tackled on an individual level. However, that is not all. The Curriculum also provides a means by which the sponsoring institution (in this case the RCGP on behalf of PMETB) can set appropriate assessments and evaluate delivery. It also has a political function, which is exercised at many levels from aiding programme directors negotiate with trusts about the requirements of posts within a general practice training programme to strategic discussions involving hundreds of millions of pounds about the necessary shift of resources from secondary to primary care. In other words:

> A curriculum is an organisational, educational, social, professional, philosophical and political statement. It is a guide to practice and a standard against which to measure the performance of the institution, its teachers its mangers and its students.[11]

A unified assessment system – the nMRCGP

Up until 2007 specialty training for general practice has been encumbered by two parallel assessment systems: Summative Assessment, a low standards,

Box 6.3 The statements of the RCGP Curriculum

Being a general practitioner
The general practice consultation
Personal and professional responsibilities
 Clinical governance
 Patient safety
 Ethics and values-based medicine
 Promoting equality and valuing diversity
 Evidence-based practice
 Research and academic activity
 Teaching, mentoring and clinical supervision
Management in primary care
 Management in primary care
 Information management and technology
Healthy people: promoting health and preventing disease
Genetics in primary care
Care of acutely ill people
Care of children and young people
Care of older adults
Gender-specific health issues
 Women's health
 Men's health
Sexual health
Care of people with cancer and palliative care
Care of people with mental health problems
Care of people with learning disabilities
Clinical management
 Cardiovascular problems
 Digestive problems
 Drug and alcohol problems
 ENT and facial problems
 Eye problems
 Metabolic problems
 Neurological problems
 Respiratory problems
 Rheumatology and conditions of the musculoskeletal system (including
  trauma)
 Skin problems

high stakes exit requirement for general practice training and the membership examination of the RCGP, a high standards, but ultimately low stakes, modular examination. Both required the passing of four components, both included a knowledge test and an examination of consulting skills and neither is linked to the current system of signing off satisfactory completion of periods of training. Happily, this situation is about to change and the new licensing examination for general practice, the nMRCGP, will bring together not only the two assessment programmes, and thus reduce the burden on trainees, but also better integrated training, learning and assessment. At the time of writing, the RCGP awaits a verdict from PMETB on its assessment proposals but is committed to a tripartite assessment comprising:

• Applied knowledge test
• Clinical skills assessment
• Workplace-based assessment.

Applied knowledge test

The applied knowledge test (AKT) will take the form of a 3-hour 200-item multiple-choice test delivered via computer terminals at around 150 professional testing centres throughout the United Kingdom. Approximately 80% of the question items will be on clinical medicine, 10% on critical appraisal and evidence-based clinical practice, and 10% on health informatics and administrative issues. All questions will address important issues relating to UK general practice and will focus on the application and understanding of knowledge rather than just the simple factual recall. Whilst candidates will be eligible to attempt the AKT at any point during their training, it is anticipated that the most appropriate point will be whilst working as a trainee based in general practice during specialty training year three (ST3).

Clinical skills assessment

The clinical skills assessment (CSA) is 'an assessment of a doctor's ability to integrate and apply clinical, professional, communication and practical skills appropriate for general practice'. The assessment is effectively an OSCE[12] (objective structured clinical examination) and builds on the College's experience with their simulated surgery assessment. The CSA will be available during a 3- to 4-week session at three points throughout the year and will take place in one location, hopefully in a purpose-built centre in London. The CSA will test a number of curriculum areas, namely primary care management, problem-solving skills, a comprehensive approach, person-centred care, attitudinal aspects and a number of practical clinical skills.

Workplace-based assessment

Workplace-based assessment is a new departure of specialty training, which in the past relied on end point assessments that had varying degrees of validity and reliability. Workplace-based assessment is a relatively recent paradigm that aims to assess those curriculum areas best tested in the workplace and to meaningfully integrate teaching, development and assessment. It is expected that workplace-based assessment will provide trainees with feedback on areas of strength and those that need development, drive learning in some important areas of competency previously poorly addressed and determine the fitness of trainees to progress to the next stage of their career.

Workplace assessment for the nMRCGP is built around a programme of evidenced reviews of progress conducted by the educational supervisor. The reviews themselves are structured around 12 clearly defined areas that have been derived directly from the core curriculum statement, *Being a General Practitioner*. The areas that workplace assessment then sets out to test are:

- *Communication and consultation skills:* communication with patients and the use of recognised consultation techniques
- *Practising holistically:* the ability to operate in physical, psychological, socioeconomic and cultural dimensions, taking into account feelings as well as thoughts
- *Data gathering and interpretation:* gathering and use of data for clinical judgement, the choice of examination and investigations, and their interpretation
- *Making a diagnosis/making decisions:* a conscious, structured approach to decision-making
- *Clinical management:* the recognition and management of common medical conditions
- *Managing medical complexity:* aspects of care beyond managing straightforward problems including the management of co-morbidity, uncertainty and risk, and the approach to health rather than just illness
- *Primary care administration and information management and technology:* the appropriate use of primary care administration systems, effective record keeping and information technology for the benefit of patient care
- *Working with colleagues and in teams:* working effectively with other professionals to ensure patient care, including the sharing of information with colleagues
- *Community orientation:* the management of the health and social care of the practice population and local community
- *Maintaining performance, learning and teaching:* maintaining the performance and effective continuing professional development of oneself and others

Box 6.4 Evidence collecting tools for workplace-based assessment

Case-based discussion
A structured discussion of a recent case based on the trainee's written record

Consultation observation tool
The consultation observation tool is used to assess and provide structured feedback on a video consultation. In secondary care consultant supervisors are instead asked to complete a mini-CEX assessment (clinical evaluation exercise)

Mini-CEX
A tool for the observation of clinical encounters or part-encounters, developed by the North American Board of Internal Medicine

Direct observation of procedural skills
A number of complex and/or intimate examinations must be observed until a mandatory section of a skills log is complete. Various optional skills may also be assessed using this method

Multi-source feedback
A simple multi-source feedback form is used for both clinician and non-clinician raters

Patient satisfaction questionnaire
Patients are also asked for their view of the doctor using a modification of the Consultation and Relational Empathy (CARE) questionnaire

Clinical supervisors' reports
A structured report is to be completed by all clinical supervisors in secondary care placements

- *Maintaining an ethical approach:* practising ethically with integrity and respect for diversity
- *Fitness to practice:* the doctor's awareness of how their own performance, conduct or health, or that of others, might put patients at risk and the action taken to protect patients.

The trainee collects supporting evidence in preparation for each review. This may be 'naturally occurring' such as events witnessed by the educational supervisor whilst in practice or through a number of structured evidence collecting tools. These evidence collecting tools are summarised in Box 6.4. Trainees must collect a minimum, specified amount of evidence before each review. All the workplace assessment tools and reviews will be completed through an electronic portfolio, to be issued to trainees on starting in training programmes.

The e-portfolio

The RCGP e-portfolio is designed to support the learning and development of the general practice specialty registrar throughout their 3-year training period and beyond into continuing professional development. The portfolio has a number of key purposes providing:

- A reflective learning log for the trainee, available to be shared (with permission) with their educational supervisor
- A record of progress towards the achievement of curricula competencies
- A repository for assessments carried out during training
- A framework for the learning agreements between learners and teachers
- A means of communication between trainees and the educational institutions that support them.

The portfolio is web-based and allows the registrar to receive automatic information, store documents and access external links such as to web-based curriculum learning support material. The portfolio will describe a learning trajectory towards the goal of independent practice, marked by the award of a Certificate of Completion of Training and a place on the GP Register.

Certificate of Completion of Training

The Certificate of Completion of Training (CCT) is the goal of specialty training. It marks the successful attainment of curricula competencies and fitness to progress to the next stage of the trainees' career, that of becoming an independent practitioner. Applications for a CCT are sent to the RCGP who then check and forward the trainees' details to PMETB, who in turn issues the Certificate. Of course, a certain amount of money, in the form of fees, changes hands along the way. The requirements of a CCT are that trainees complete a prescribed programme of training and satisfy its assessment requirements. However, there is another way. Applicants who believe that they have undertaken training equivalent to that of a CCT programme in general practice (e.g. applicants from countries with similar training programmes to those in the United Kingdom) can submit a structured portfolio of their experience to the PMETB under Article 11. PMETB, advised by the RCGP, will then decide whether or not to issue a Statement of Eligibility for inclusion in the GP Register.

Summary

The year 2007 marks a turning point in the training of general practitioners and whilst there remain some outstanding issues to resolve such as finding the funding for increased time in primary care, expanding training capacity without compromising quality and rationalising contractual arrangements there is much cause for optimism. The curriculum is an excellent foundation and is already assisting deaneries in the design of fit for purpose posts and programmes. There have been sensible reforms to selection and assessment systems and we now have a system of supervision linked, for the first time, to the destination specialty. But have we got it right?

General practice is rapidly changing as the National Health Service struggles to hold itself together under the entropic forces of privatisation and the future for the specialty is uncertain. Roles and responsibilities are dissipating in relatively uncontrolled ways, performance related pay has focused the energies of practices on achieving financial targets and competition from the private sector is mounting. The curriculum lays down a marker, but like all such documents it is a political instrument of its time and whilst undoubtedly the immediate future for general practice training is better than it ever has been, quite how long the reforms to specialty training remain 'fit for purpose' remains to be seen.

Further information

The full text of the RCGP Curriculum and information about all the nMRCGP assessments can be found at www.rcgp.org.uk.

References

1 Sibbett C, Thompson W, Crawford M, McKnight A (2003) Evaluation of extended training for general practice in Northern Ireland: qualitative study. *British Medical Journal* **327**: 971–973.

2 Bowler I, Swanwick T (2005) Extended training in general practice: senior general practice registrars in the London Deanery. *Education for Primary Care* **16**: 34–40.

3 Piele E, Gallen D, Buckle G (2003) *Higher Professional Education for General Practitioners*. Oxford: Radcliffe.

4 Department of Health (2003) *Modernising Medical Careers*. London: Department of Health.

5 Department of Health (2002) *Unfinished Business: Proposals for the Reform of the SHO Grade*. A Report by Sir Liam Donaldson, CMO for England: Department of Health.

6 Patterson F, Lane P, Ferguson E, Norfolk T (2001) Competency based selection system for general practitioner registrars. *BMJ Career Focus*. http://careerfocus.bmj. com/cgi/content/full/323/7311/S2-7311 (Accessed 10 May 2007).

7 Royal College of General Practitioners (2007) *Guidance on the Content of Specialty Training Programmes in General Practice Intended to Lead to the Award of a CCT*. London: Royal College of General Practitioners. www.rcgp.org.uk/certification_/ certification_home/certificate_of_completion_of_t/the_cct_training_programme_-_f.aspx (Accessed 10 May 2007).

8 WONCA Europe (2002) *The European Definition of General Practice/Family Medicine*. Amsterdam: WONCA Europe.

9 General Medical Council (2001) *Good Medical Practice*. London: General Medical Council.

10 Royal College of General Practitioners (1972) *The Future General Practitioner: Learning and Teaching*. London: Royal College of General Practitioners.

11 Grant J (2006) Principles of curriculum design. In: Swanwick T (ed.) *Understanding Medical Education*. Edinburgh: Association for the Study of Medical Education.

12 Boursicot KAM, Roberts T, Burdick WP (2007) Structured assessments of clinical competence. In: Swanwick T (ed.) *Understanding Medical Education*. Edinburgh: Association for the Study of Medical Education.

Chapter 7 **Royal College of General Practitioners**

Nav Chana

What is it?

The Royal College of General Practitioners (RCGP) is the academic organisation in the United Kingdom for general practitioners. In actual fact, the term 'college' is a bit of misnomer. The RCGP does not have students or lectures in the traditional sense. Instead the word refers to a medical institution, which encourages professional development through a network of approximately 30,000 GPs. Unlike the British Medical Association (BMA), the RCGP does not act as a trade union for its members. The BMA might focus on negotiating pay and terms and conditions for GPs, but the RCGP's primary focus is to encourage and maintain the highest standards of general medical practice and act as the 'voice' of general practitioners on education, training and standards issues. In the short history since its foundation in 1952 the RCGP has played a part in achieving some significant milestones, including the establishment of vocational training in general practice.

The RCGP has a federal structure and operates through local college branches (known as faculties) and a central council. There are currently 31 faculties in the United Kingdom, one in the Republic of Ireland and another one for overseas members. Every member and associate member is automatically allocated to membership of one of the faculties of the college. Faculties mirror the organisation of central council, which is the governing body and key decision-making arm of the college. Each faculty is run by a faculty board and at least one representative from each faculty sits on the college council. Membership of the council includes additional 'officers' other than those nominated through the faculties so that representation is reflective of the needs of general practice.

Choosing General Practice: Your Career Guide. Edited by Anne Hastie and Anne Stephenson. © 2008 Blackwell Publishing, ISBN: 978-1-4501-7070-3.

The RCGP is a membership organisation. Whilst the standards of general practice are promoted for all GPs, membership of the RCGP enables access to a number of RCGP initiatives.

What does the RCGP do?

The RCGP has stated its views on the benefits of membership[1] as follows:
1 Standards for the whole profession
2 Improving the quality of care for patients
3 Sharing with other GPs
4 Learning and development
5 Making a difference
6 Information and knowledge.

Each of these will now be explored in more detail.

Standards for the whole profession

One of the ways the RCGP has shown its commitment to developing standards has been the publication of the new RCGP curriculum.[2] This is a competency-based curriculum, which has been developed following an extensive literature review and is presented as a series of 15 curriculum statements. These statements signpost the key areas for teaching, learning and assessment in general practice.

Probably the most relevant statement to those considering a future in general practice is the first curriculum statement: *Being a General Practitioner*.[2] As an illustration, this statement defines six key domains, which underpin the entire curriculum. The first three relate to the primary care consultation:
1 Primary care management
2 Person-centred care
3 Problem-solving skills, specific to general practice

The remaining competencies are more complex and consider requirements for learning beyond the consulting room:
4 A comprehensive approach
5 Community orientation
6 A holistic approach.

These domains are key to developing the requisite attributes of generalism. The curriculum is set out in a manner which enables close articulation with the RCGP's assessment framework.

Standards for certification

For most trainees the most direct contact with the RCGP's standards will come from the RCGP assessment framework. From August 2007, all new entrants to specialty training programmes for general practice will undertake a new integrated assessment system for certification. This will be mandatory for doctors to obtain a certificate of completion of training (CCT) enabling entry to the General Medical Council's GP register and for membership of the RCGP. The assessment system, currently designated as nMRCGP, will consist of three modules, each of which has to be satisfactorily completed. The modules are:

• An applied knowledge test (AKT)
• A clinical skills assessment (CSA)
• A workplace-based assessment (WPBA).

Each assessment draws its assessment blueprint directly from the RCGP curriculum. The new assessment framework replaces one of the existing routes to membership, currently known as the MRCGP examination, which is widely known and internationally regarded as a high-quality postgraduate examination. Although it is being phased out, the intellectual property generated will be retained as nMRCGP takes over.

Standards for recertification

With the requirement for certification comes the need for recertification of established GPs. The RCGP is actively involved in developing standards for recertification which are drawn from the curriculum and will form part of a process for recertification for all GPs on a regular (five-yearly) basis. This will become an essential requirement of revalidation as set out in the recently published white paper: *Trust, Assurance and Safety – The Regulation of Health Professionals in the 21st Century.*[3]

Standards for established GPs

The RCGP has an assessment framework for established GPs who have not undertaken the membership examination. For these GPs, membership by assessment of performance (MAP) is the alternative route to membership. MAP reproduces the standards nested within the current MRCGP examination and relies on the generation of a portfolio of evidence that established GPs collate, leading to an assessment by external assessors.

Fellowship is the highest form of membership that an individual can attain within the college. Members of five continuous years can self-nominate based on their experience in one, any or all of six achievement categories designated as follows:

1 Clinical practice
2 Patient-centred practice
3 Leadership
4 Teaching and education
5 Innovation and creativity
6 Academic and research.

These reflect the breadth of activity in the discipline of general practice. Independent experts review the portfolio of information contained within the categories against stated criteria.

Improving the quality of care for patients

The RCGP has a number of schemes specifically designed to improve patient care. Setting the standards for individual GPs has already been described above, but the RCGP has also developed initiatives which enable organisations to achieve quality standards that improve the quality of care provided for patients. There has been much talk of 'kite-marks' for general practice organisations. Currently such schemes are voluntary and the RCGP accredits organisations against published criteria leading to awards such as the Quality Practice Award[4] or Quality Team Development.[5]

Sharing with other GPs

General practice can sometimes be a lonely place to work. For many GPs, especially those working in rural communities, networking with other GPs can be difficult. Peer support through the RCGP faculty structure is one way in which GPs from different practices can come together and share best practices. Most RCGP faculties organise meetings and events specifically for this purpose. Each faculty hosts an annual general meeting where new members are elected to join the faculty board. The Board meets regularly to discuss college business and key issues and is an excellent way for GPs to get involved with the college.

Learning and development

Lifelong learning is an important attribute contributing to the professional competency of GPs. The RCGP organises a series of professional and scientific meetings throughout the year, which are designed to contribute to the process of continuing professional development. These include national and regional courses, conferences and study days. Such events are discounted for members who can also benefit from accessing a raft of e-learning resources. Listed below are some examples of programmes, distance learning qualifications and learning packages offered by the RCGP to its members.

Programmes
- The RCGP substance misuse unit offers a programme leading to a certificate in substance misuse.
- The RCGP leadership programme is designed to develop leadership skills both in the NHS and other work environments.

Distance learning
- The RCGP Learning Unit[6] is a collaborative venture between the RCGP and the University of Bath. They produce distance learning packages primarily for GPs, which may also be suitable for nurse practitioners and practice nurses.
- The RCGP in collaboration with the University of Dundee offers a Postgraduate Certificate in Medical Education for General Practitioners.[7]
- The Masters in Primary Healthcare in Relation to Secure Environments (PHIRSE)[8] is a generic educational programme for healthcare professionals in the United Kingdom. It is a collaborative venture with the University of Lincoln and the Trent Multi-Professional Deanery.

Educational packages
- The *RCGP Learning Guide*[7] for professional development is a resource designed to help, support and encourage the professional development of a general practitioner.
- The PEP (Phased Evaluation Programme) e-KIT[9] is a new online learning product designed to identify educational needs. The original PEP programme has been used by trainers and trainees alike to define the learning needs for trainees at the start of the training programme.

Influencing the future and getting involved
Increasingly, politicians and civil servants are heavily influencing the NHS and for many GPs engaging with these political issues is now more important than ever. It is emerging more clearly that the future of primary healthcare requires both effective clinical leadership from GPs, and effective engagement with many stakeholders including providers of care, managers and politicians. Given that the RCGP is constantly asked for its position relating to issues affecting primary care, the College can provide opportunities for grass roots GPs to influence the future. Getting involved with the RCGP can happen at many levels. Accessing local faculties has already been discussed but there are many opportunities to join working groups, clinical guideline development groups and clinical networks.

RCGP working groups
The RCGP has many currently active working groups and members are welcome to join to contribute to debates and help develop policy in these key areas. Below are just some of the currently operational working groups:
- Health Inequalities Standing Group
- Health Informatics Standing Group
- Rural Practice Standing Group

- Sex, Drugs and HIV Task Group
- Mental Health Task Group
- Adolescent Task Group
- Disability Task Group.

Developing clinical guidelines

The RCGP has a number of guideline development groups and members with an interest or expertise in key areas are welcomed to join the groups or review documents generated by the groups.

RCGP clinical networks

The RCGP Clinical Network facilitates best practice across all the areas in which clinical groups are involved. The network welcomes approaches from members who would like to become involved in its activities, have any comments or questions, or would just like more information on what is happening in this expanding area of the college.

Becoming a commentator

Members can shape the College's response to consultations each year and the RCGP involves as many members as possible in this work. In this capacity, members are asked to comment on clinical topics, practice issues, regulatory matters, ethical and medicolegal issues and many areas of public policy where they impact on GPs.

Information and knowledge

Accessing the relevant information at the right time is increasingly important for busy GPs. The RCGP offers an extensive informatics service. Most familiar will be the *British Journal of General Practice* (BJGP), which is the RCGP's flagship academic journal, published monthly. However, there are many other informatics services provided by the college:

1 Enquiry and Literature Search Services: An enquiry service answering queries, which can provide information on all aspects of general practice except financial, contractual and legal issues. (These latter issues probably better dealt with by the BMA.)
2 Databases (available from RCGP web pages) include:
   - Guidance for GPs which links to published documents for GPs.
   - An acronym finder.
   - Contact information for NHS organisations and staff. This is useful for providing contact lists for mail-merge purposes to target a product or event to a particular sub-group within the NHS (e.g. PCT Clinical

Governance Leaders or Practice Managers in London, etc.). Contact and profile information on all UK members of parliament can also be provided.

3 The college library: The Library stock includes a unique reference collection of MD and PhD theses from general practice, an international selection of primary care journals, and a loan collection of College publications. The Library Catalogue contains material that traces the evolution of general practice and primary care within the National Health Service, and contains many articles, reports and books by members of the College.

4 Information sheets: A series of documents, which act as a short introduction to some of the key issues surrounding general practice. They are accessible through the website.

5 Fact sheets: A set of articles that cover topical and specific areas in primary care.

6 Summaries: A collection of papers, which summarise important documents relating to general practice including reports, consultation documents and policy statements released by the government and other bodies.

7 News services:
- Seven Days[10] provides weekly summaries of important events, developments and guidance in primary care. This can be read on the website or can be requested electronically.
- The RCGP e-bulletin[11] is a bi-monthly email bulletin with College activities, news and events and is sent to approximately 30,000 doctors.

Becoming a member

Associate membership

For many GPs in training the first contact with the RCGP will be after registration with the RCGP Certification Unit, which will automatically provide associate membership. Associate membership may also be held by trained GPs who have not pursued full membership but wish to retain links with the College. Associate membership confers academic benefits (such as access to the BJGP) and enables networking opportunities, but further development and influencing of RCGP policy is only available to full members.

Full membership

Full membership confers all the membership benefits specified above. There are two full membership routes:

- Sitting the membership examination, which will be the route for all doctors seeking certification from August 2007
- Membership by Assessment of Performance (MAP) designed for practising GPs who have not taken the membership examination.

The future of general practice

The future of general practice is bright, but there are significant challenges that lie ahead. These include the need to prevent the fragmentation of care, to achieve the correct balance between generalism and specialisation, to maximise the quality of doctor–patient interaction, and to maintain the highest possible standards of professionalism. The RCGP in setting out its aspiration to 'encourage, foster and maintain the highest possible standards in general practice' is ideally placed to secure the future of general practice.

Acknowledgement: The author would like to thank the RCGP for providing the information for this chapter.

References

1 Royal College of General Practitioners. *Have You Got It.* http://www.rcgp.org.uk/pdf/Have%20you%20got%20it.pdf
2 Royal College of General Practitioners. *Being a General Practitioner.* http://www.rcgp.org.uk/PDF/curr_1_Curriculum_Statement_Being_a_GP.pdf
3 Department of Health (2007) *Trust, Assurance and Safety – The Regulation of Health Professionals in the 21st Century.* London: HMSO.
4 Royal College of General Practitioners. *The Quality Practice Award.* www.rcgp.org.uk/quality_/quality_home/quality_practice_award.aspx
5 Royal College of General Practitioners. *Quality Team Development.* www.rcgp.org.uk/quality_/quality_home/qtd.aspx
6 Royal College of General Practitioners Learning Unit. www.bath.ac.uk/health/rcgp
7 Royal College of General Practitioners. *RCGP Learning Guide.* www.bath.ac.uk/medicalupdates/learning-guide/index.htm
8 Trent Multiprofessional Deanery. *Masters in Primary Healthcare in Relation to Secure Environments (PHIRSE).* www.trentdeanery.nottingham.ac.uk/general/prison.htm
9 Royal College of General Practitioners Scotland. *PEP eKIT.* http://www.rcgp.org.uk/councils_faculties/rcgp_scotland/products_services/ pep_ekit.aspx
10 Royal College of General Practitioners. *Seven Days.* http://www.rcgp.org.uk/information_services/information_services_home/information_services_publicati/seven_days.aspx
11 Royal College of General Practitioners. *RCGP e-bulletin.* http://www.rcgp.org.uk/information_services/information_services_home/is_publications/e_bulletin.aspx?page = 499

Chapter 8 **Further training opportunities**

Steve Mowle

Introduction

Fifteen years ago newly qualified GPs had largely two job options, either to become a locum GP and work sessions in different practices, or to apply to become a partner. Job opportunities since then have widened significantly for newly qualified GPs. In some areas innovative primary care organisations (PCOs), educators and GPs joined forces to organise salaried doctor schemes, which typically offer 1- to 2-year contracts to help bridge the path from GP registrar to becoming either a salaried GP or a GP partner. The schemes were particularly developed in areas where recruitment and retention were a problem and the earliest schemes occurred in South London and the East of England. One such example is the vocationally trained associate (VTA) scheme, which is discussed below describing the various components of a scheme.

A new general medical services contract (nGMS)[1] was introduced in 2004 and the recruitment opportunities for new GPs appear to have declined with many applicants applying for individual GP posts that are advertised. At such a time, cash strapped PCOs might divert funds towards more pressing priorities, although undoubtedly over the next 10 years with increasing numbers of doctors retiring[2] it is highly likely that the number of these schemes will significantly increase in number. The other major advantage of joining this type of scheme is that it enhances a new GP's curriculum vitae (CV) and makes him or her a more attractive employment option, particularly if specialist skills have been acquired.

The author of this chapter moved from Cardiff, where he was an Academic Research Fellow, to London. The move was facilitated by joining the VTA scheme in 1999 and allowed the acquisition of local knowledge, which

---

Choosing General Practice: Your Career Guide. Edited by Anne Hastie and Anne Stephenson. © 2008 Blackwell Publishing, ISBN: 978-1-4501-7070-3.

resulted in him joining a practice as a partner the following year. This experience afforded the author a view of both academic practice and inner city general practice in two non-training practices within 2 years of completing his vocational training scheme.

History of the VTA scheme

The vocationally trained associate scheme is one of the oldest and most established salaried schemes in the country. It was set up by the South London Organisation of Vocational Training Schemes (known as SLOVTS) in Lambeth, Southwark and Lewisham (LSL) in 1994.[3] The priorities of the scheme were to give newly qualified doctors a positive experience of working in inner city general practice while providing support and additional training. In addition to this the associates would support stressed, inner city practice GPs at a time of change or development. The VTA scheme's working week was as follows:

- Seven sessions working in two busy inner city practices
- One session for a facilitated, peer group meeting
- One session for an individual project, research or audit presentation
- One session for personal and professional development.

The scheme was initially funded by London Initiative Zone grants, allocated as part of extra money available to primary care in London following the Tomlinson Report.[4] Subsequently mainstream funding was allocated by the Health Authority and complemented by contributions from practices.

The VTA scheme has been incorporated into the Salaried Practitioner Programme (SPP), which includes the benefits of the former salaried academic GP programme at King's College, London. This now offers a choice of sessions to young GPs including a clinical speciality or academic attachment in teaching, research or a Masters in primary health care. The SPP GPs' work is divided into:

- Clinical sessions in general practice
- One to two sessions per week in a clinical speciality or academic attachment
- One session per week in a peer support or self-directed learning group.

The bulk of the Salaried Practitioner Programme costs are now covered by the practice which pays a contribution for the clinical sessions and the local PCO which pays for the support structures and specialty placements.

Ingredients of a Salaried GP Scheme

Suitable clinical placement

The GP placement needs to be in a practice where the salaried GP can further develop. The practice should not be under stress or disorganised so that it can provide a safe environment for a newly qualified GP. Practices therefore need to be carefully selected, preferably with the input of local clinicians and the PCO's locality management.

Ideally the salaried doctors should be able to select the practice where they undergo their clinical attachment. Under the VTA scheme the associates were central to the practice allocation process. The associate GPs selected practices by arranging visits to potential practices and then negotiated with their fellow associates, who at that stage were strangers. This was a powerful way to start working within a group.[5]

Peer support groups

This is central to most salaried doctor schemes whereby members of the scheme meet regularly. Usually it is a strongly self-directed process by which the group decides it own structure and function. As this is a contracted part of the working week each group member has a responsibility to contribute and influence the way the group works.

The group can often provide very significant support to its peers by solving problems and confronting issues within their practice. In addition, the groups often include topic-based discussions as well as guest speakers and social events. In addition to the regular meetings some schemes also offer a residential, which further allows the group to bond into a cohesive support structure. Ideally the residential should be early in the programme.

Historically, these self-directed support groups have spawned further young practitioner groups, which continue beyond the duration of the scheme and further underline the value placed on these groups by the participants.

Clinical specialty attachments

Many salaried GP schemes offer the opportunity to develop an area of clinical specialty. This can range from a half day to two full days spent either in a community specialty or within a hospital specialty. Clearly there is the potential for a wide variety of different specialties to choose from and those being favoured are often dermatology, family planning, community child health, drug and substance misuse management, cardiology and public health. Over the course of the programme, a diploma could also be achieved, for example the Cardiff Diploma in Dermatology.

Care should be taken in selecting a specialty that is not only of interest to the GP but also has some possibility of success in using those skills within the locality where the GP wishes to settle. For example, in one borough in South London there are already a number of GPs with a special interest in dermatology as well as three major teaching hospitals with large dermatology departments all fighting for a small number of patients.

Academic attachments

In some of the salaried doctor schemes, it is possible to undertake an academic attachment and develop teaching skills, research skills or undertake a master's degree in primary health care. This is an ideal opportunity for GPs early in their careers to have a significant academic taster and decide whether this is a career pathway they would like to follow.

Most master's programmes require between 2 and 3 days of part-time study and this should be considered when applying for the degree as a high level of commitment is required to finish the course. Some academic programmes are more flexible and after 1 year would result in a postgraduate certificate and after 2 years of study would result in a postgraduate diploma. These academic attachments also allow for vital networking in their chosen field, which can often lead to involvement in larger research projects and ultimately to a career in academic general practice.

Mentoring

Most salaried GP schemes ensure that all participants have a named mentor who is there to ensure that the salaried GP is well supported within the practice. The scheme should ensure that the mentoring occurs within protected time and is a condition of the contract between the practice and the salaried GP. All scheme members should be encouraged to formulate a personal development plan (PDP) with their mentors and this could form the focus of a periodic evaluation on how well the GP was progressing through the year. Some mentors are experienced GP trainers, but most are non-trainers. The mentoring time is often a two-way process in which the mentors may feel they have gained at least as much as they gave to their mentee.

Scheme coordinator

The scheme coordinator may either be someone from an educational background or a GP, and both have their pros and cons. In an ideal scheme, members should be able to appreciate how powerfully the group can self-direct and support each other without having an expert clinician to give all the answers. On the other hand, the GP facilitator may be able to offer a deeper insight into the clinical experiences of the group members than the educationalist.

Elective

A minority of schemes allow for a paid elective of 2–3 months, which can be a very attractive option and might mitigate working in less desirable practices or short-term attachments.

Pay, terms and conditions

The salaried GPs may be employed by the local PCO or the GP practice where they work. They should have a fixed term contract of between 1 and 2 years and pay is generally in line with the lower end of the scale for salaried GPs. There may be a study leave budget attached to the scheme and medical defence subscriptions may also be covered by the scheme.

Care should be taken to ensure that maternity leave arrangements are clear from the outset, both for the scheme member and the employing practice or PCO. It may be possible for scheme members to take their maternity leave and return to the scheme either at the same practice or a similar one locally. Contracts should be broadly in line with the British Medical Association's (BMA) recommendations for a salaried GP contract.

Some schemes allow part-time working but this can be problematic for scheduling the peer support group and specialty attachment. This would leave only a small time (two to three sessions) for the clinical attachment, which may not be regarded as being very good value for money by the practice or PCO. However, PCOs should be aware that it is likely that the future workforce will want to work flexibly and factor this in when designing a scheme.

Summary

Salaried GP schemes are an attractive option for GPs who wish to further develop their skills within a supportive framework. Although they are usually aimed at newly qualified GPs these schemes could also be used to attract established GPs who wish to refresh their skills or move to a new part of the country where the job has a built-in support structure. These schemes are more likely to thrive in areas where there are recruitment and retention problems.

The experience in South London is such that a large number who went through the VTA scheme remained in South London as principals or salaried doctors. Indeed this high quality scheme still attracts a good number of applicants. Support and professional development are essential ingredients to achieving a successful salaried GP scheme which will attract and retain high calibre applicants.

References

1 Department of Health (2005) *Standard Medical Services Contract*. London: Department of Health.

2 Mathie A G (2000) *The Primary Care Workforce: An Update of the New Millennium.* London: Royal College of General Practitioners.
3 Hughes J (2006) Learning Initiatives in primary care across South East London: implication for recruitment and retention of GPs. *Work Based Learning in Primary Care* 4: 152–155.
4 Tomlinson B (1992). *Report of the Inquiry into London's Health Service, Medical Education and Research.* London: HMSO.
5 Harrison J, van Zwabenberg T (eds) (2002) *GP Tomorrow*, 2nd edn. Oxford: Radcliffe.

Chapter 9 **Flexible training and working**

Anne Hastie

Introduction

Over the last few decades there has been increasing pressure from doctors of both sexes to improve their work/life balance. White male doctors no longer dominate the profession and traditional ways of working will not be able to deliver the future service required by the National Health Service (NHS) for the benefit of patients. *The NHS Plan*[1] in 2000 was closely followed by a consultation document *A Health Service of all the Talents: Developing the NHS Workforce,*[2] which identified the need for investment and reform within the NHS. The Department of Health (DH) acknowledged the need for flexible working environments for doctors at various stages of their careers.[3] This became part of the consultation to develop the NHS workforce with an emphasis on flexible training and working in order to make the best use of the wide range of skills and knowledge available. In 2004 responsibility for employment issues and promoting the NHS as an employer was devolved to NHS Employers.

Further changes will be required in the working patterns of doctors in training, including redesigning services to minimise night work.[4] Opportunities for flexible working after completion of training are equally important and financial constraints must not be used as an excuse for preventing change in working patterns. In fact, new ways of working are even more important when funding is limited to ensure a high standard of healthcare delivery.

Background

The number of women working in medicine has increased every decade since the introduction of the NHS in 1948 and it is predicted that women doctors will outnumber men by 2012.[5] Economic factors mean that many

Choosing General Practice: Your Career Guide. Edited by Anne Hastie and Anne Stephenson. © 2008 Blackwell Publishing, ISBN: 978-1-4501-7070-3.

more women continue to work after becoming parents and the high divorce rate in Britain has not escaped the medical profession, placing a financial burden on both partners. Men and women who are seeking a better work/life balance are demanding part-time and flexible ways of training and working. This has been supported and encouraged by the DH through their Improving Working Lives initiative.[6]

Between 1950 and 1973 women were admitted to medical schools on a restricted quota system. In 1973 the Sex Discrimination Act was introduced so the restricted quotas had to be abolished and by 1992 women had achieved parity in the numbers of medical school entrants. The year 1990 saw reduced hours of work for junior hospital doctors to 72 hours and the European Working Time Directive (EWTD)[7] will reduce this to 48 hours by 2009. However, these hours remain excessive for many women and some men.

Allen[8-10] extensively researched factors affecting women doctors, attracting a lot of attention from the medical profession and the DH. Her research showed that in 1986 only 3% of women doctors (and no men) were in part-time training posts although one-third were considering it in the future and there was a definite imbalance between supply and demand for part-time training. At the same time only 4% of women doctors were in part-time career posts although 97% thought there should be greater availability, especially of job-sharing opportunities. Allen's research indicated the need for a radical reassessment of the medical career structure and the way it was structured with more opportunities for flexible training and working.

Davidson, Lambert and Goldacre[11] followed the career destinations of doctors who qualified in 1977, and Lambert and Goldacre those who qualified in 1988.[12] They showed that 7 years after qualifying in 1988, 53% of women working in general practice and 20% in hospital specialties worked part-time. Eighteen years after qualifying in 1977 the number of doctors working part-time in general practice was similar at 51% but the number of women working part-time in hospital specialties had risen to 42%.

Forty-eight percent of doctors (24% male and 74% female) who qualified in 1995 indicated that they might wish to work part-time at some point in their career[13] and one of the challenges will be making this a reality. Full-time work remains the norm with a higher degree of status in comparison to some part-time arrangements. Although women are the main gender wanting to work flexibly there is an increasing demand from men, which may have helped contribute towards a greater acceptance of new working patterns.

There has been a long-standing concern about medical workforce planning, which is complex and has had a fragmented approach in the past[2] and these studies highlighted the need for medical workforce planning to take into account the whole time equivalent years of work. The number of women doctors shown not to be working in these studies is significantly less than that in other professions,[14] but the high cost of training means it is worth trying to retain these doctors. Developing flexible ways of working should help recruit and retain more GPs.

Flexible training

Flexible training was first introduced in the 1970s in order to retain doctors who would otherwise have left the profession. Flexible training, or Less Than Full-Time (LTFT) training as it is known in Scotland, provides a means to work less than full-time for a group of doctors who represent a valuable NHS resource for future service provision. New flexible training funding arrangements for hospital doctors were introduced in June 2005[15,16] to reflect the increasing demand for part-time training. In the future trusts will need to look innovatively at their rotas in order to incorporate flexible training as the new arrangements require every trust to have 20% of their trainees working flexibly within 5 years, subject to demand.

Who is eligible for flexible training?

Flexible training is accessible to doctors in training who have a well-founded reason for being unable to work full-time. In practice, the majority of flexible trainees are women and men who wish to look after their young children for part of the week, and there are a small number who are carers for other family members. Also eligible are doctors with physical or mental health problems, who would like to continue their training but are unable to do so full-time. The national guidance on eligibility for flexible training is that Category 1 applicants are automatically eligible and take priority for funding over Category 2.

Category 1
• Parents of young children who wish to spend part of the week at home
• Doctors caring for sick or dependent relatives
• Doctors who are unable, for health reasons, to work full-time.
Recent parliamentary legislation (Employment Act 2002 part IV) imposed a legal obligation on employers to give reasonable consideration to a request for part-time working by any employee with a child under 7.

Category 2
• Doctors wishing to train part-time, while in paid employment for the remainder of the week
• Doctors wishing to train part-time in order to follow non-medical interests.

In recent years deaneries have had to restrict flexible training to Category 1 applicants because they have not had sufficient funding for both categories.

Certificate of Completion of Training (CCT)

The framework for general practice training is now defined by the Postgraduate Medical Education Training Board (PMETB) under Article 10 of the Order.[17] General practice trainees must do at least 3-year full-time training or equivalent part-time within a 7-year period preceding their application for a CCT.[18]

The GP training programme must include:
- 12 months' full-time equivalent in an approved training practice with an approved GP trainer
- 12 months' full-time equivalent in other specialties approved for GP training
- 12 months' full-time equivalent in combinations of the above.

It is hoped in the future that at least 18 months' full-time equivalent will be spent in general practice but this will be subject to available funding. In most cases training is provided by a 3-year GP specialty training programme although there may be a few shortened schemes for doctors making a career change providing their previous experience can count towards their GP training.

Recruitment to GP training

Doctors who wish to train flexibly should check their eligibility with the relevant deanery and then apply through the national recruitment process in the same way as those wishing to train full-time. Everyone who is involved in assessing applicants is trained under equal opportunities and will not be told that the applicant plans to train flexibly. If an applicant is successful and offered a GP specialty training programme they should then confirm their wish to train flexibly. Deaneries will give guidance on organising flexible training but a placement is subject to an employer willing to employ the doctor on a flexible basis and the individual doctor is responsible for organising their flexible training placement.

GP flexible training in secondary care posts

Flexible training enables doctors to reduce their working week but the exact proportions favoured can vary between deaneries although the majority of flexible trainees work 60% of full-time. Flexible trainees have traditionally been supernumerary employees and deaneries have contributed to their basic salary costs. However, as the budget for flexible training is one of a number competing for funding, it may be insufficient to meet all demands for flexible training. This has resulted in deaneries and trusts looking at other ways to promote flexible training.

Flexible training in hospitals is not an easy option and takes time to organise. It is particularly difficult for general practice training as trainees rotate through several specialties. The local postgraduate deanery will give guidance but it is the responsibility of the flexible trainees to organise their flexible training. Even though a trainee has been successfully selected for a GP specialty training programme it is still up to the hospital trust whether they are prepared to employ him or her flexibly. However, all employers must seriously consider requests to work less than full-time and must give good reasons if they say no.

The EEC directive for the training of GPs requires trainees to work at least 1 week full-time during the hospital component of their training.[19] A good week to choose is the first week of one of the posts, when the hospital and departmental induction is taking place. The rest of the training must be at least 50% of full-time. Many deaneries will only fund flexible training up to 80% and expect those who want to work more than 80% to work full-time. New flexible training arrangements ensure that pay for a hospital flexible trainee is proportional to the full-time pay.[15] The employing trust and not the deanery fund any out of hours (OOHs) payments.

The timetable of the flexible trainee should be based on the full-time timetable of trainees in the same grade and the same department.[16] All parts of the post should be done at the same agreed percentage:
• Daytime work
• Educational activities
• On call
• Out of hours.

A maximum of 6 months' training can be completed without OOHs in special circumstances. Doctors who are breastfeeding are exempt from OOHs but they need to check that this will not affect the educational approval of their post.

Types of flexible training posts

Slot shares

The deanery already funds 50% of full-time posts approved for GP training. Each slot sharer can work more than five sessions and the deanery can choose to fund the additional costs over the normal full-time post. For example, if two slot sharers work 80% each (160% in total) the deanery can choose to fund the additional 60%.

Supernumerary posts

For supernumerary posts the deanery funds the daytime sessions worked e.g. five sessions for 50% flexible trainees, six sessions for 60%, etc. and the trust funds the additional costs associated with any additional hours of actual work and the OOHs supplement. Some deaneries will only fund five or six sessions.

Reduced sessions in a full-time post

Full-time posts are already 50% funded by the deanery even if no one is in post. If a department has an unfilled full-time post then this should be used instead of a supernumerary placement.

Educational approval

If flexible trainees are working as a slot share or part-time in a full-time post educational approval should already be in place. However, if a supernumerary post is being created using flexible training funding educational approval must be obtained on an 'ad personum' basis before starting in post. This will require the submission of details of the post to PMETB by the Director of Postgraduate General Practice Education (DPGPE).

- A completed PMETB Form B (GP)
- Personal development plan (PDP) for the post
- Clinical timetable
- Educational timetable, including attendance at the VTS half-day
- Name of the educational supervisor
- Percentage of full-time.

   Provisional educational approval is granted by the DPGPE and ratified by the Deanery GP Education and Training Committee (or equivalent). PMETB is the statutory body that gives formal educational approval.

Part-time training in general practice

The budget for funding registrar posts in general practice is the same for full- and part-time posts, unlike hospital training where there is a separate budget for flexible training. A placement is subject to a GP trainer willing to employ a part-time registrar but this is rarely a problem as practices like having a doctor who will be with them for more than 1 year. Training as a registrar can be on a 'non-continuous' basis subject to approval by the DPGPE.

   Registrars must work at least 50% of full-time and work at least 1-week full-time during their general practice placement.[19] The timetable should be based on what a full-time registrar works in the same practice. The regulations require a part-time registrar to work the same percentage of clinical sessions, educational sessions, on call and OOHs. The registrar cannot reduce the number of clinical sessions but continue with a 100% of educational activities. At the end of their part-time training period they should have completed the same amount of training as a full-time registrar.

One session equates to 4 hours and a full-time working week comprises 10 sessions, which equates to 40 hours per week plus OOHs (pro rata for part-time). A typical full-time registrar timetable might include:
• Seven clinical sessions
• One session to attend a group educational half-day programme
• One flexible, planned, individual educational session
• One session for a tutorial.

The timetable will vary according to local arrangements, e.g. if there is a weekly educational full-day, but it is important that registrars get sufficient clinical experience. Although a session should be 4 hours it is recognised that some sessions may be longer while others shorter, but the overall full-time working week should be 40 hours plus OOHs. Registrars and trainers should therefore look at the total workload/hours rather than the hours of an individual session.

GP specialty training programme directors prefer registrars to attend their educational half-day (or day) programme every week to avoid disruption. A part-time registrar could choose to attend every week for a year and then do other activities for the remainder of their training. If they want to continue going to the educational programme after a full year it should be at the expense of other educational activities e.g. the flexible session. For example a registrar working 50% might choose to go to the educational programme during term time and have the flexible session during the academic holidays. Some degree of flexibility around educational activities is acceptable providing it is at the appropriate percentage and supports the registrar's learning needs.

Calculations of time required to complete the equivalent of full-time training

Percentage worked (%)	Part-time training for a 12-month full-time post (months)	Part-time training for a 6-month full-time post (months)
50	24	12
60	20	10
75	16	8
80	15	7.5
100	12	6

Absence during training

The regulations allow up to 1 week of leave during a 6-month period of training for sickness, maternity, adoption and paternity but the absence in excess of this must be made up by extending the GP registrar contract. During a 3-year GP training programme intermittent absences that add up to 6 weeks (pro rata for shorter periods of training) will not normally be expected to be made up. If the absence is for a longer time it must be made up but not necessarily in the specialty or post where the absence occurred.[19] DPGPEs can use their discretion if absences exceed the guidelines by a small amount. In many cases it is possible to extend the registrar contract during the general practice placement to cover relatively short absences during hospital training. Trainees need to check with the RCGP/PMETB that their plans to make up lost time comply with the regulations.

Flexible working as a GP

Once a doctor is qualified as a GP the opportunities for part-time and flexible working become increasingly common and varied. Flexible working does not necessarily mean part-time and to be truly flexible a post should include annualised hours. GPs now have the opportunity to work in a variety of ways (e.g. partnership, salaried, locums) and a variety of associated disciplines (e.g. teaching, research, management).

Forty years ago many full-time male GPs thought their part-time female colleagues were working for 'pin money' and part-time pay was proportionately less than full-time. A partnership in general practice was considered a job for life and GPs were eyed with suspicion if they tried to move jobs. In addition, the workload of the 'junior partner' was often greater than the 'senior partner' and it could take many years to reach financial parity. This has gradually changed and there is now much greater fairness in practices. Approximately 20% of GPs who are currently partners work part-time[20] and the trend is for this to increase.

Part-time partnership

A partnership is the traditional way of working as a GP. Partners are self-employed and receive a share of the profits rather than a salary. Individual practices choose how to apportion shares according to workload and this is usually based on the number of clinical sessions worked per week but should also take into account other responsibilities such as:
• Practice management
• Information development

- Staff development
- Clinical governance lead
- Teaching, e.g. GP trainer, undergraduate teacher
- Appointments outside the practice.

In some cases part-time partners can organise flexible working e.g. only working during school term time. This can work well if there is an older partner who would like to work full-time during the school holidays but wants extra time off during the school term in order to travel when holidays are cheaper.

Sessional GPs

This group includes most GPs who are not partners. Locums are self-employed but all other sessional GPs are salaried. Being a salaried GP is a popular way of working part-time and these GPs are employees of the practice. Their salary has to be negotiated with the employing practice and is usually proportional to the number of sessions worked, but may be significantly less than a GP partner who has the additional responsibility of running the practice. The BMA provides a model contract for salaried GPs[21] and doctors should seek help if they are unhappy with the terms and conditions of the post on offer. The normal hours of work for a full-time salaried GP are 37.5 hours made up of nine sessions of 4 hours and 10 minutes, and part-time would be pro rata.

Doctors who only want to do a limited amount of work may be eligible for the GP retainer scheme,[22] where the GP is salaried but also supernumerary and this is described in more detail in Chapter 10. Locum work has its advantages as the GPs can choose when they want to work and they can now be part of the NHS pension scheme. However, there are significant disadvantages such as no employment rights and loss of NHS continuity of service after 12 months. Meeting the criteria for revalidation may also become a problem in the future.

Portfolio GP (See chapter 12)

Many GPs now have a portfolio career, which means having more than one job and in some cases several jobs, which fit together to make a whole. GP partners may have a portfolio career but choose to put all their earnings into the practice partnership, from which they receive a share of the profits and a typical full-time timetable might include:
- Six sessions working as a GP
- One session working as a hospital practitioner

- Two sessions working as a GP specialty training programme director
- One weekly half-day
- One monthly OOHs.

Alternatively a GP may have two separate jobs with completely separate income streams such as:

- Six sessions as a GP
- Four sessions as an associate director in a postgraduate deanery.

Teaching and training

Once the domain of the full-time GP it is now increasingly popular for part-time GPs to become involved in teaching and training. It is even possible to be the GP trainer of a full-time registrar providing the trainer ensures that the registrar has appropriate cover when the trainer is not working. Teaching undergraduates is very popular with part-time GPs as it is not as demanding on their time as being a GP trainer. Alternatively they could be the educational supervisor of a GP retainee or GP returner.

Sabbaticals

Working as a doctor in the NHS is demanding even if one opts to work part-time. Once an individual is appointed as a GP, he or she may stay in the same practice for 20 or more years. A sabbatical can allow a period of recreation or the opportunity to develop new professional skills. In addition younger doctors may wish to take time out between jobs to pursue other interests, travel or work abroad.

Organising a sabbatical takes time and motivation with many obstacles to overcome but the benefits can be considerable to the individual, his or her family, colleagues and patients. There are several ways in which a GP can take a sabbatical including:

- Unpaid leave
- Paid leave
- Prolonged study leave
- Gaps between jobs.

Prolonged study leave (PSL) is probably the most financially generous way of taking a sabbatical in the NHS and is unique to general practice. It provides GPs with the opportunity to develop knowledge and skills in an area of personal career interest. However, funding is dependent on availability in their local Primary Care Trust and in times of financial constraint funding may not be approved.

Pensions, maternity leave and other benefits

It is very important that part-time GPs are fully aware of the rules and regulations of NHS benefits to help them plan their future, including retirement. GPs who have worked part-time or have portfolio careers may need specific help with their financial planning. Many older GPs have regretted not sorting out their NHS pension appropriately and some younger GPs have missed out on maternity pay because they did not read the regulations. The NHS provides GPs with very good benefits under the General Whitley Council Conditions of Service.[23] The conditions are regularly updated and further changes are inevitable, as the Department of Health would like all doctors to be covered by conditions that have been agreed for other NHS employees.

NHS pension

The NHS pension scheme has many benefits, which are protected. Pension difficulties for workers in the private sector or those with personal pensions have highlighted the advantages of public sector pensions. No one is too young to be thinking about a pension and the earlier a pension is started the better the benefits on retirement. GPs are recommended to stay in the NHS pension scheme and the few who have opted out have often regretted their decision. Actuaries have assessed the benefits of the NHS pension scheme as being worth approximately 20% of overall pay.[24]

GPs are pensioned under the practitioner method, which is based on career average earnings. The pensionable pay for each year of membership is uprated to the pay levels in force when the practitioner stops paying contributions and this is known as dynamising. If a GP has some hospital or other NHS officer membership the Pensions Agency will automatically assess whether it is possible and beneficial to convert to a practitioner pension for all work or give a separate pension for the officer work. Practitioner membership cannot be converted to a final salary pension and the rules are complex, see www.nhspa.gov.uk

Maternity leave

Maternity leave legislation was amended as a result of the Employment Act 2003 and implemented from 6 April 2003.[25] Most NHS medical staff are covered by the General Whitley Council agreement, which is more generous than Statutory Employment Law. Registrars working in general practice are employed by their GP practice and not the NHS but there is an agreement that they are entitled to similar maternity leave and pay as in the Whitley agreement for other trainees. Salaried GPs should ensure that their contract has a continuity clause to cover previous NHS work before joining their current practice. The regulations are complex and individuals should seek help from the British Medical Association if their employment record does not allow full entitlements.

Other benefits

The NHS provides a range of other benefits for GPs, many of which are covered by the General Whitley Council conditions of service.[25] Although local alternatives can be agreed upon they should be at least as favourable and most NHS employers continue to use national terms and conditions. These include:
- Ill health retirement
- Life assurance and family benefits
- Redundancy
- Adoption leave
- Paternity leave
- Parental leave

Summary

The demand for flexible training has increased and it needs to become mainstream rather than supernumerary. Flexible trainees should not be seen as different but just another way of working and it should be possible to move in and out of full-time training. Hospitals are reviewing the way their trainees work because of the EWTD and MMC, which creates the ideal opportunity to incorporate and mainstream part-time training.

General practice is an excellent career for doctors who want to work part-time and/or flexibly. Supply and demand for GPs has meant that many practices have had to be creative in the way they employ their GPs if they want to recruit and retain good doctors. However, this is a two-way process and GPs need to be realistic in their demands and take into account the needs of their colleagues. The glass ceiling is less of a problem in medicine than other professions and this is particularly true for general practice. Many part-time GPs have achieved success in high office, academic general practice, medical politics and management.

References

1 Secretary of State for Health (2000) *The NHS Plan – A Plan for Investment, A Plan for Reform.* London: Department of Health.

2 NHS Executive (2000) *A Health Service of All the Talents: Developing the NHS Workforce.* London: Department of Health.

3 Department of Health (2002) *Improving Working Lives for Doctors.* London: Department of Health.

4 NHS Modernsing Agency Hospital at Night (2003) www.modern.nhs.uk/hospitalatnight

5 Griffiths E (2003) Just who are tomorrow's doctors? *BMJ Careers* **326**: 4.

6 Department of Health (2001) *Improving Working Lives Standard.* London: Department of Health.

7 Department of Health (2003) *The European Working Time Directive, Guidance.* London: Department of Health.

8 Allen I (1988) *Doctors and Their Careers.* London: Policy Studies Institute.

9 Allen I (1992) *Part-Time Working in General Practice.* London: Policy Studies Institute.

10 Allen I (1994) *Doctors and Their Careers: A New Generation.* London: Policy Studies Institute.

11 Davidson JM, Lambert TW, Goldacre MJ (1998) Career pathways and destinations 18 years on among doctors who qualified in the United Kingdom in 1977: postal questionnaire survey. *British Medical Journal* **317**: 1425–1428.

12 Lambert TW, Goldacre MJ (1998) Career destinations seven years on among doctors who qualified in the United Kingdom in 1988: postal questionnaire survey. *British Medical Journal* **317**: 1429–1431.

13 British Medical Association (2001) *BMA Cohort Study of 1995 Medical Graduates, Sixth Report.* London: BMA.

14 Parkhouse J (1991) *Doctors' Careers.* London: Routledge.

15 NHS Employers (2005) *Doctors in Flexible Training: Equitable Pay for Flexible Medical Training.* Leeds: NHS Employers.

16 NHS Employers (2005) *Doctors in Flexible Training: Principles Underpinning the New Arrangements for Flexible Training.* Leeds: NHS Employers.

17 Postgraduate Medical Education and Training Board (2003) *The General and Specialist Medical Practice (Education, Training and Qualifications) Order.* London: The Stationery Office.

18 Royal College of General Practitioners (2005) *PMETB Certificate of Completion of Training.* London: RCGP.

19 Joint Committee on Postgraduate Training for General Practice (2004) *A Guide to Certification.* London: JCPTGP.

20 Department of Health (2002) *General Practitioner Recruitment, Retention and Vacancy Survey 2002 England and Wales.* London: Government Statistical Service.

21 British Medical Association (2003) *Model Terms and Conditions of Service for a Salaried General Practitioner Employed by a GMS Practice.* London: BMA.

22 NHS Executive (1998) *GP Retainer Scheme. Health Service Circular 1998/101*. Leeds: Department of Health.
23 Department of Health (2004) *General Whitley Council Conditions of Service*. London: Department of Health.
24 NHS Pensions Agency (2004) *A Guide to the NHS Pension Scheme*. Fleetwood: Department of Health.
25 Department of Trade and Industry (2003) *Maternity Rights*. London: DTI.

Chapter 10 **Returner and retainer schemes**

Anwar Khan and Rebecca Viney

Introduction

People may choose to take career breaks for various reasons. Retainer and returner schemes for general practitioners (GPs) provide supportive and educational working environments, which help retain or encourage doctors to return to general practice.

The number of women working in medicine has increased every decade since the introduction of the National Health Service (NHS) in 1948. It is predicted that women doctors will outnumber men by 2012 and 70% of GP registrars are already women. The European Working Time Directive has been one of the most important changes to benefit doctors and improve their working lives, although working hours are still excessive for many doctors.

Recent parliamentary legislation imposed a legal obligation on employers to give reasonable consideration to a request for part-time working by any employee with a child under 7 or who is a carer. It is increasingly easy to find part-time work as a salaried GP, which facilitates the maintenance of clinical skills and enjoyment of patient contact without the burden of partnership responsibilities. However, those GPs with heavy domestic responsibilities may temporarily need protected posts with a strong emphasis on education.

This chapter will explain the returner and retainer schemes, including recent changes and their advantages and disadvantages.

Returner schemes

Research has shown that 20 years after qualification almost a quarter of doctors are not working in medicine.[1] Doctors who are qualified GPs leave the specialty for a variety of reasons including domestic commitments and other

Choosing General Practice: Your Career Guide. Edited by Anne Hastie and Anne Stephenson. © 2008 Blackwell Publishing, ISBN: 978-1-4501-7070-3.

career pathways.[2,3] The most common reasons for not working in a substantive general practice post include[3]:

- Domestic and non-medical work
- Working abroad
- Pharmaceutical industry
- Public health
- Other clinical specialties
- GP locum or private GP
- GP retainer scheme
- Retirement.

Doctors who have been away from general practice for a significant amount of time appreciate the provision of a re-entry course, as they often lack confidence to return to clinical work.[4–6] The workforce crisis in primary care was acknowledged[7] a decade ago but it was not until the new millennium, that the recruitment and retention of GPs became a national priority. The NHS Plan[8] required the appointment of an additional 2000 GPs into substantive posts by 2004 and one of the most cost effective methods of increasing the number of GPs in the workforce was to recruit doctors who had left the specialty.

In November 2002, the Department of Health launched a National Returner Campaign, which included the introduction in England of the GP Returner Scheme to facilitate a re-entry programme into general practice through refresher training.[9] The campaign was aimed at qualified GPs in the following circumstances:

- GPs working as locums rather than in substantive NHS posts
- GPs who were not working
- GPs who were working but not in general practice.

The returner scheme was designed to encourage doctors back into general practice by giving them a period of refresher training after a career break. The pace of change in the NHS has been rapidly increasing since 1990 and the returner scheme provided a secure environment to ease GPs back into the NHS.

Burton and Jackson promoted work-based learning in primary care[10] and extending work-based learning to doctors wishing to return to general practice through the GP Returner Scheme offered an opportunity to refresh skills within general practice, rather than just attending courses. Learning in the workplace was felt to be an essential part of refresher training, in order to restore the confidence of these doctors and to enable them to gain clinical experience. It also allowed these doctors to become part of the primary healthcare team and learn in a multidisciplinary environment.

The scheme provided a maximum of 6 months' full-time or equivalent part-time refresher training with an educational supervisor who was usually a GP trainer. The training provided returning GPs with a supportive environment in which to refresh their professional skills and ensure the quality of their work through regular formative assessment. The content, format and length of training were tailored to the needs of the individual.

Funding

The GP Returner Scheme was funded by the Department of Health and administered by NHS Professionals, enabling deaneries to support GPs who wished to return to the workforce. However, funding for the scheme and administrative support from NHS Professionals was withdrawn after only 3 years at the end of 2005.

The withdrawal of central funding resulted in deaneries finding a variety of options such as self-funding, funding from primary care trusts (PCTs) or deanery funding. The GP Retainer Scheme can be a suitable alternative for experienced GPs who have only been out of practice for a few years. The concept of self-funding produced a dialogue between the British Medical Association (BMA) and Department of Health as the legality of working unpaid is complex. It could also seem discriminatory to ask GPs to self-fund as the majority are women.

The introduction, at PCT level, of the GP Performer List in 2004 made it more difficult for doctors to return to general practice after a prolonged career break. Most PCTs now require a GP who has been out of practice for more than 2 years to undergo a period of refresher training and/or work in a supervised environment before he or she is fully included on the PCT's Performer List. Revalidation may add to the problem and returning to practice might be impossible without a returner scheme. It would be a considerable waste if this resulted in good enthusiastic GPs lying fallow.

Current schemes

Doctors interested in returning to general practice apply to their local postgraduate deanery where they are invited for an informal interview to discuss their individual circumstances. Prior to the introduction of the GP Returner Scheme deaneries only had a very small number of doctors returning to general practice each year. Since then numbers have increased significantly and applications are continuing at a steady pace. It is probable that the increasing emphasis on flexible working has attracted some of these doctors back to the NHS, who had left because of the previous rigidity of employment within medicine.[11] As a result of this demand some deaneries have developed an infrastructure to assess and support GP returners. Deaneries can also use the same scheme for the induction of European Union (EU) GPs, on the basis that they have never been in clinical practice in the United Kingdom.

A regulatory framework exists, which stipulates those doctors who are eligible to work in general practice. Doctors are eligible to work in general practice in the United Kingdom in the following circumstances:

- Hold a Joint Committee on Postgraduate Training for General Practice (JCPTGP) certificate of prescribed or equivalent experience.
- Hold a Postgraduate Medical Education Training Board (PMETB) Certificate of Completion of Training (CCT) if training is finished after 30 September 2005.
- Have a legal exemption to holding a JCPTGP or PMETB certificate.
- Have acquired rights to work in general practice (in some circumstances this only enables the doctor to work as a locum or assistant).

Each deanery will have developed its own system of assessment before accepting a doctor onto the scheme and this may include:

- Formal interview
- Knowledge test, e.g. multiple choice questions (MCQ)
- Simulated surgery
- Self-assessment, including confidence rating scales
- Learning needs assessment.

On completion of the scheme the doctor needs to be in a position to satisfy the PCT that he or she can be admitted on to their Performer List without conditions. It is for the respective PCT to determine whether to admit the doctor to their Performer List and under what conditions. The deanery has an advisory role with the PCT and the doctor but no power to compel.

As mentioned earlier, individual deaneries have variations of the scheme and this chapter will describe the London Deanery as an example. London had the largest number of GP returners[12] in England and has developed an Induction and Refreshment Scheme for UK and EU GPs. The aim of the scheme is to:

- Attract UK qualified GPs back into general practice.
- Offer a suitable induction and adaptation programme to EU GPs who would like to continue their GP career in the United Kingdom. These doctors have a legal right to practice in the United Kingdom, providing they have an appropriate GMC certificate.

Applicants must be resident in London and indicate their intention to work in a substantive NHS GP post in London for at least 2 years (or the equivalent part-time) following their refresher training. This may not necessarily be completed immediately following their refresher training, e.g. maternity leave.

The deanery needs to ensure these GPs (whether qualified from United Kingdom or European Union) are fit for purpose to work as independent general practitioners and the needs of each GP will be different. Many UK returners will feel unsure about how competent they are to practice and the majority will require a period of refresher training. EU GPs require a period of adaptation to a different health care system. The initial assessment process is not only aimed to select those who would benefit from an induction into general practice but also to produce an 'educational prescription', which identifies their learning needs.

The length of the GP Induction and Refreshment (UK/EU) programme is up to 6 months full-time or equivalent part-time. This may be shortened following the individual learning needs assessment, in agreement with the deanery and the GP. Doctors may work in another field of medicine or in a non-medical career at the discretion of the Director of Postgraduate General Practice Education (DPGPE) while undergoing refresher training.

Appointment processes

Before acceptance on to the programme the doctor has an interview with the associate director responsible for the scheme. The assessment process includes an interview, MCQ paper and a simulated surgery. A specific language assessment may be used if the doctor is not a native English speaker.

A pass in the MCQ is required before attempting the simulated surgery and a maximum of two attempts are allowed. The total scores in the MCQ and simulated surgery are used for ranking purposes in the event of there being more candidates than available funded placements. A pass in the assessments is valid for a year and if for any reason a placement is not found these will have to be re-taken.

Interview

The discussion is a two-way process giving the doctors an opportunity to talk about their intentions and enables the associate director to find out more about the individuals and the support they may require. Factors needing to be identified and discussed include:
- Curriculum vitae
- Length of their break in service
- Expectations of their return
- Country of GP training and previous experience
- Level of confidence and current knowledge
- Perceived learning needs
- Where and when the doctor would like to work
- Whether they want to work full-time or part-time, where full-time is nine sessions per week.

Multiple choice papers

After their interview the applicant will be asked to sit a MCQ paper. The purpose is to satisfy that the doctor's basic medical knowledge has been kept up to date and that the GP is able to read and write medical English for general practice. The pass mark is dependent on the individual paper. (there are a number of peer-referenced versions of the test.) A maximum of two attempts are allowed.

The paper consists of a variety of multiple choice questions, which include true/false answers, single-best answers or a number of questions of the extended matching variety. The questions cover topics that a new doctor would be expected to be able to answer and are aimed at undergraduate finals level.

Simulated surgery

The applicant will be asked to attend a simulated surgery providing they pass the MCQ paper. The simulated surgery assesses clinical competencies including communication, history taking and clinical assessment. The simulated surgery is not primarily a test of knowledge but that of consulting and communication skills.[13] The simulated surgery is intended to be like an everyday surgery in any general practice – a real morning or afternoon surgery. The patients are role players who are fully trained to present themselves as real patients and the cases are typical general practice problems. An observer accompanies each role player and plays no part in the consultation but looks at the consulting skills, making observations on a written schedule. These observations allow personal feedback to be given to candidates after the simulated surgery. The areas of consulting skills tested are as follows:
- Gathering medical information
- Eliciting the patient's concerns
- Explaining the diagnosis
- Managing the problem
- Closing the consultation.

These assessments help inform the deanery about the refresher training requirements of the doctor as well as forming part of the selection procedure.

Task list prior to placement

Once a doctor is offered a place on the GP Induction & Refreshment Scheme (UK and EU), there are a number of tasks that must be completed with the London Deanery and the relevant PCT. GPs cannot begin their placement unless these tasks have been completed:

- Criminal Records Bureau (CRB) check
- Occupational health – a confidential health questionnaire needs to be completed
- Original documentation of the following items:
  ◦ GMC registration
  ◦ Medical Indemnity Insurance
  ◦ Certificates relating to qualifications
  ◦ Passport (Birth certificate is not acceptable.)
- References – two are required and one must be a clinical reference but relatives or friends cannot provide a reference.

GPs are initially put on the PCT Performer list with the following conditions:
- Successful completion of the GP Induction & Refreshment Scheme
- Obtaining two UK references during their placement.

Finding a suitable placement

The deanery will assist the doctor in finding a suitable placement appropriate for their individual circumstances and in the majority of cases this will be in a training practice. Some GPs who have only been out of practice for a short period of time may not need to be placed within a training practice. In these cases the deanery may exercise its discretion about a suitable environment, e.g. a practice working towards training accreditation.

Successful applicants are referred to the local trainer group convenor and where possible these doctors are placed in practices that do not have a current GP registrar. If this is not possible a practice can have more than one learner at the discretion of the associate director, providing they have the appropriate accommodation and educational capacity. Doctors joining the scheme must make themselves available to visit potential practices and to be interviewed by the trainer. A placement is subject to a trainer being willing to employ an individual applicant.

Deaneries are not permitted to become involved with individual pay negotiations and it is up to the PCT to set the returner's salary. The PCT reimburses the practice:
- An agreed salary negotiated between the PCT and doctor
- A trainer's grant – the supervising trainer is paid a grant in order to provide the appropriate training during the induction period.

Teaching the returner

The educational supervisor is usually an approved GP trainer and non-trainers must have appropriate experience of teaching and training. Clearly the educational supervisor has a valuable and crucial role in helping the returners achieve the most from their placement, by ensuring that the teaching is individualised to the returners' particular needs and by encouraging them to develop the skills of lifelong learning. A successful placement will be invaluable in ensuring the smooth return of these crucial members of the general practice workforce of the future. The returners should be encouraged to develop a personal development plan (PDP) at an early stage.

The induction programme uses a number of different learning methods, which include:

- Lectures and expert presentations
- Group discussions
- Working with different health care professionals to understand what they do and how they work
- Peer group and communication skills sessions
- Video, role-play and simulated surgeries for further developing communication skills
- Clinical work under supervision in general practice
- Tutorials with their GP mentor and other members of the primary healthcare team
- NHS logbook
- Hands on computer experience
- English language sessions as appropriate
- Regular appraisals.

Formative assessments

There are a variety of formative assessment tools used[14] and include the following:

- The simulated surgery assessment is useful to identify some of the learning needs, particularly around communication skills.
- Self-assessment confidence rating scale.
- NHS logbook.
- Use of videos of consultations – the value of the use of video cannot be overemphasised as the consultation is the cornerstone of general practice.
- Learning needs generated by direct patient contact. This is an excellent way of identifying learning needs as they arise and not letting the moment pass without action.
- Joint surgeries with a trainer are a fruitful source of learning needs although patients may find it hard to ignore the fact that a more experienced and more familiar doctor is in the consulting room. It helps if the patients are told in advance the nature of the joint surgery.

End point assessment

Doctors joining the scheme have already fulfilled the certification require-ments and are not required to pass the end stage assessment, which is es-sential for those completing GP specialty training. However, the London Deanery requires doctors to give evidence of successful completion of their placement by returning the structured NHS log book (completed by their mentors) at the end of the placement as well as undertaking an 'exit' simu-lated surgery. These tools enable the deanery to advise the PCT that the GP is fit for independent practice and the conditions on the Performer List may be removed. The doctor receives a certificate of successful completion of their placement.

An exit interview gives the deanery feedback on the scheme with suggestions for improvement. In addition, the interviewer should discuss with the returner their future career intentions, educational needs and other issues.

The GP Retainer Scheme

The original Doctor Retainer Scheme was introduced in 1969. Although the concept was inspired and far ahead of its time, it had severe limitations and only allowed doctors to work a maximum of two sessions a week in general practice. Education and employment rights were not included and these GPs frequently became deskilled, lost confidence and many never successfully returned to independent general practice. In June 1998, the new GP Retainer Scheme was introduced, which is more flexible and allows doctors to work up to 52 sessions per quarter in general practice. This can be combined with a limited amount of non-general medical services work, which is usually limited to a maximum of two sessions.

The retainee should have well-founded personal reasons for only under-taking limited paid employment and the DPGPE will take individual cir-cumstances into account when deciding whether to accept a doctor onto the scheme. The scheme is not intended for those doctors who are committed to a career in another area, such as GP academics. Nor is it appropriate for a GP who chooses to only work a few sessions per week, for example when their children are at full-time school.

The Department of Health published detailed guidance[15] and the British Medical Association produced a model contract. This has been further im-proved to include generous amounts of protected time for education, incor-porating the minimum terms and conditions allowable for salaried GPs under the new general medical services (GMS2) contract.[16]

The practice

GP registrar ST3 training practices meet the criteria for hosting a retainer scheme GP. However employment of a retainee will need to be approved by the deanery in order to ensure that the educational element of the scheme is appropriate and the needs of the retainee are met.

Non-training practices may be approved for employing a retainee and will usually be visited by the deanery. A named educational supervisor should undertake preparation of the practice and themselves for supervising and employing a retainee.

The practice should:
- Provide a sufficiently wide range of services
- Provide adequate induction
- Provide named educational supervisor
- Help and give advise to the retainee during clinical sessions
- Notify the deanery of any changes in premises, partnership or employment/educational arrangements of the retained doctor.

The practice must offer the retainee one session of continuing professional development (CPD) for every eight clinical sessions worked and a retainee working only one session a week is entitled to a minimum of eight sessions of CPD per year. Retainees should be allowed leave to attend CPD activities, or if it occurs at a time when not normally working they can take time off in lieu.

The educational supervisor

A named GP, who works regularly within the practice, should be appointed as the retainer's educational supervisor. The rules of the scheme also require that a named clinical supervisor should be available during clinical sessions to provide help and advice, debrief at the end of sessions, and discuss dilemmas and interesting cases if required. In most cases the same person fulfils both the educational and clinical supervisor roles but if the educational supervisor is not available during the retainer's clinical sessions the practice must nominate another suitable person as clinical supervisor.

Protected time should be made available for the educational supervisor and GP retainee to meet on a regular basis at a mutually convenient time for tutorial, feedback, case discussion or other aspects of general practice that the retainee feels is needed.

The duties of the educational supervisor

Approval to be an educational supervisor will require that the supervisor is competent and committed to the role. The following 'competence and commitment' has been adapted from the work by Dr Vik Mohan and colleagues at the Peninsula Institute.

Competence
The educational supervisor should be able to demonstrate his or her:
* Ability to write a learning needs analysis
* Ability to write a personal learning plan
* Understanding of the principles of adult learning
* Understanding of the different learning styles, be aware of his or her own preferred learning style and be able to explain the implications of this
* Knowledge of the range of learning resources available.

The educational supervisor should have acquired these core competencies via formal educational training and/or experience in an educational role. If no training/experience can be demonstrated then the prospective educational supervisor must make an undertaking to attend a course at the earliest opportunity.

Commitment
The educational supervisor should:
* Provide dedicated, regular educational supervision, in protected, mutually convenient time. One notional hour per month would be a reasonable minimum standard.
* Invite the retainee to practice-based events in protected time, such as practice meetings, in-house training, away-days, and significant event meetings.
* Ensure the workload of the doctor takes into account that this is a supported, developmental post and that all members of the practice are aware of this.

Evidence of the above should be included in structured feedback from the retainees. In London the educational supervisors are invited to the deanery twice a year to explore the aims of the scheme and share best practices. The meeting explains the 'nuts and bolts' of the Department of Health guidance to those who are new to the scheme and provides a forum for sharing ideas and answering questions.

Additional educational opportunities for the GP retainee

Self-directed learning groups
Many deaneries have nurtured and supported the development of self-directed learning groups (SDLGs) over the past decade and these groups have gone from strength to strength. They are invaluable in supporting GPs who have become professionally isolated and are also an information resource via e-mail and their websites for doctors who might otherwise be out of the loop.

Away-days

Many deaneries bring their retainees together at regular intervals so they can learn together and explore how to make the most of the scheme from each other's experiences.

Newsletters

It is important that opportunities to develop new skills and changes in the NHS effecting GPs are conveyed to these doctors. E-mail has facilitated the sharing of relevant information, via newsletters, which are greatly valued by the doctors on the scheme.

Sessions

The minimum number of sessions that may be worked per week is one session and the maximum is 52 per quarter (usually spread evenly throughout the period as four sessions per week). The weekly quota of sessions may be increased or decreased by mutual agreement. However, one session a week is felt to be too little to maintain clinical skills over a prolonged period of time and many deaneries will only approve this as an interim measure.

A session for salaried GPs, including retainees, is defined by the BMA as 4 hours and 10 minutes. However, if it suits their individual circumstances the GP retainees may work in fractions of a session, e.g. 3 or 5 hours. This includes administrative time and dialogue with the educational supervisor/clinical supervisor at the practice. The retainees may agree to home visits and on-call responsibility providing this is completed within the agreed sessional time and is in accordance with the agreed educational plan as well as fitting in with their domestic responsibilities.

The retainees may also work up to two sessions a week of additional work outside of the practice with the prior approval of the deanery, for instance as clinical assistants, out of hours (OOHs) workers or as GP tutors. The retainees must notify their defence organisation of any additional work.

Length of time on the scheme

The maximum length of time on the GP Retainer Scheme is usually 5 years and there is no age limit to joining the scheme, providing there is an intention to return to a career in general practice. Retainees are approved to be on the scheme for a year at a time and they must apply annually to be re-approved. Family commitments are by far the most frequent reason given for being on the scheme and in the past the 5-year time limit was very unpopular. Retainees commented that it took longer than 5 years before the youngest child reached school age[17] but employment law has changed since the scheme was introduced. The BMA lawyers have advised that while it is legally understood that fixed term contracts such as the retainer scheme can exist, the consequences of having a fixed term contract and being employed for 1 year or more means that an employee may be entitled to full employment rights.

After 5 years on the scheme, most practices are now keeping their retainees in their practice as either salaried GPs or new partners. Under the old GMS contract there was little flexibility for the practice to offer part-time employed positions. The new GMS contract, introduced in 2004, has removed the financial disincentives of replacing partners with salaried doctors and hence a practice can now use its budget to retain valuable members of the team.

The 5-year time limit does give some protection against producing a long-term ghetto for women GPs. However, in exceptional circumstances and at the discretion of the DPGPE the scheme may be extended for a year at a time to an absolute maximum of 10 years.

Payments

The practice is reimbursed £59.19 (2006/2007) for every clinical and educational session and whilst the retainee is on leave including annual leave, maternity, paternity, adoptive, sickness, an emergency involving a dependent or other pressing family reasons. The reimbursement is intended to offset some of the costs to the practice of employing the GP retainees and supporting them in their educational needs.

Doctors on the GP Retainer Scheme are entitled to a fixed annual sum as a contribution towards their professional expenses, which in 2006/2007 was £310. This is paid as a lump sum by the deanery at the beginning of the scheme and on an annual basis thereafter as long as the GP remains a member of the scheme. Tax and National Insurance are deducted at source, but the allowance is not superannuable. Defence organisations have a reduced charge for retainees and doctors should contact their organisation for precise up-to-date costs. Indemnity for all additional work, other than the GP retainer sessions, must be discussed and agreed with the medical defence organisation on an individual basis.

Contractual Issues

Retainees are by definition employees and it is a statutory requirement for an employee to have a contract of employment. The BMA's new model contract for the GP Retainer Scheme[16] is in line with the minimum terms and conditions of employment for salaried GMS GPs. Some deaneries require any practice employing a GP on the retainer scheme to use the BMA's new model GP retainer scheme contract, which must be unchanged. This ensures parity and equity for all retainees and avoids a postcode lottery of contracts.

Summary

GPs increasingly wish to take a career break from general practice and the GP Returner Scheme has been an important and successful initiative to increase the recruitment of GPs. The total cost to the Department of Health for a GP to undertake the maximum 6 months full-time on the scheme is considerably less than the cost of 3 years of specialty training to produce a new GP.

An evaluation of the scheme after the first year of implementation enabled initial difficulties in establishing the programme to be readily addressed.[12] The finding that returning GPs in London successfully obtained permanent posts on completion of the course demonstrates the value of the programme.[18]

The GP Retainer and Returner schemes are vital to ensure doctors who take a career break or only have a limited clinical input, due to childrearing or other personal reasons, have the support to rebuild their confidence in a safe clinical environment.

References

1 Goldacre MJ, Lambert TW, Davidson JM (2001) Loss of British-trained doctors from the medical workforce in Great Britain. *Medical Education* **35**: 337–344.

2 Baker M, Flett A, Williams J (2002) The work commitments of British general practitioners: a national survey. *British Journal of General Practice* **50**: 730–731.

3 Hastie A, Clark R (2005) The GP Returner Scheme: the London Deanery experience of the first 50 applicants. *Work Based Learning in Primary Care* **3**: 23–30.

4 Baker M, Williams J, Petchey R (1995) GPs in principle but not in practice: a study of vocationally trained doctors not currently working as principals. *British Medical Journal* **310**: 1301–1304.

5 Baker M, Williams J, Petchey R (1997) Putting principals back into practice: an evaluation of a re-entry course for vocationally trained doctors. *British Journal of General Practice* **47**: 8l9–822.

6 Baker M, Batstone G, Kisely S (1998) Returning doctors to medicine. *British Medical Journal* **316**: S1–S2.

7 Mathie T (1997) The primary care workforce crisis: a time for decisive action. *British Journal of General Practice* **47**: 3–4.

8 Secretary of State for Health (2000) *NHS Plan – A Plan for Investment, a Plan for Reform.* London: Department of Health.

9 National Health Service (2002) *General Practitioners – Returning to the NHS.* London: Department of Health.

10 Burton J, Jackson N (eds) (2003) *Work-Based Learning in Primary Care.* Oxford: Radcliffe.

11 Vaughan C (1995) Career choices for Generation X. Young doctors want flexible career paths, not long term commitments. *British Medical Journal* **311**: 525–526.

12 Hastie A (2004) The GP Returner Scheme. *Education for Primary Care.* **15**: 501–504.

13 Burrows P, Khan A, Bowden R, Jackson NJ (2004) The fresh start simulated surgery. *Education for Primary Care* **15**: 328–335.

14 Khan AA, Naish J (2004) Learning needs assessment. In: Jackson NJ, Carter Y (eds) *Refugee Doctors.* Oxford: Radcliffe.

15 NHS Executive (1998) *GP Retainer Scheme.* Health Service Circular 1998/101. Leeds: Department of Health.

16 British Medical Association (2005) *Model GP Retainer Scheme Contract.* London: BMA.

17 Hastie A (2002) Assessment of the GP Retainer Scheme. *Education for Primary Care* **13**: 233–238.

18 Hastie A, Clark C (2005) The GP returner scheme; the London experience of the first 50 applicants. *Work Based Learning Journal.* **3**: 23–30.

Chapter 11 **Principals, partnerships and salaried posts**

Rebecca Viney and Catherine Jenson

Introduction

There are two main ways of undertaking a substantive career in general practice. One is to be self-employed either in partnership with others or on a single-handed basis, and this type of work has historically been described as being a 'principal'. The other main option is to be salaried, which means being employed by a practice or primary care organisation (PCO). Both types of GPs are now titled 'performers' as they actively provide direct medical care and must gain a place on a PCO performer list in order to work as a GP. Principal GPs are additionally termed 'providers' which describes their role in managing a service.

In the past GPs sought a partnership or a single-handed practice after completing their training and there were few options to work in any other way other than a locum. A principal post was usually full-time, with out-of-hours and on-call responsibilities, and for life as it was rare for a doctor to change practice.

Recent years have seen many drivers that are changing this traditional way of working. These include an increasing proportion of women doctors, changing social trends towards a work/life balance, new national legislation for equal opportunities, disability discrimination, flexibility, part-time workers[1] and NHS Improving Working Lives standards.[2] Two other significant drivers have been the change in employment law such that employees gain employment rights after 12 months and the new General Medical Services (GMS) contract which allows practices to recruit additional salaried doctors when partners leave without the financial disincentive of the previous GMS contract. Part-time contracts are increasingly common and there are also increasing opportunities for GPs to take on work outside their surgeries including clinical work in

---

Choosing General Practice: Your Career Guide. Edited by Anne Hastie and Anne Stephenson. © 2008 Blackwell Publishing, ISBN: 978-1-4501-7070-3.

areas of special interest, medical education, research and leadership. GPs can use these opportunities to build a career that best suits their personality and individual circumstances.

The factors described above are making salaried work increasingly popular. Indeed, it is now the preferred initial type of work for newly qualified GPs and the particular benefits of salaried posts will be described in this chapter. There is also a trend for fewer practices to advertise partnership vacancies when a partner leaves, which means there are fewer opportunities to enter a partnership than in the past. The reasons for this will be explored in this chapter.

GP principals and partners

What is a GP principal?

A GP principal is traditionally a GP with his or her 'own' list of patients, working in a self-employed capacity as an 'independent contractor' to provide general medical services for the patients. In the most recent NHS reforms, patients are registered with a practice rather than individual GPs so this definition is now only appropriate for single-handed GPs.

GP partners

GP principals working together traditionally form partnerships. A partnership can be defined as 'the relationship which subsists between persons carrying on a business in common with a view of profit'.[3] It may come as a surprise to lay readers that the majority of GPs are still working in this way, running a business for profit rather than being employed by the NHS. However, in practice they are managed by primary care organisations (PCOs) who pay for the services carried out and (increasingly) monitor the quality of the work done.

Types of partner

As well as working single-handed and within the traditional pattern of partnership, it is also possible for GPs to be in partnership with people who are not GPs, such as practice managers and nurses. Any partner is 'joint and severally liable' which means the partners share responsibility for their own and each other's actions. This requires a high degree of trust and is a responsibility that not all GPs are willing to take, hence the popularity of salaried posts. This is also an important reason why it is still relatively rare to find a nurse or manager in partnership with doctors.

Non-profit-sharing partners

Some practices offer GP posts as non-profit-sharing partners. In effect they are salaried posts but the 'partner' title results in additional responsibility for the management and quality of the staff and services offered. Such posts may also lack the benefits of a salaried contract (see below under 'Salaried GPs'). In a profitable practice these posts are likely to be less financially rewarding than a profit-sharing partnership and often for equivalent work. However, they can have a guaranteed income level which can be attractive in certain situations. For example, if the practice is about to incur large expenses by rebuilding their premises, or if the GP's own situation is uncertain and they cannot make the long-term commitment to the partnership that profit-sharing requires. In general it is strongly recommended that such partnerships are considered with caution as they may mean the new partner has the same workload and responsibility but without the profit. Some would say all of the pain without the gain.

Differences between being a partner and salaried

Many new partners, whether full- or part-time, find it difficult to understand the implications of being self-employed and no longer having the 'rights' of an employee. In some ways partnership is like a marriage and requires work and effort, with give and take on both sides. The partnership contract is a vital legal document that determines the terms and conditions for the partners and should be agreed upon before joining a partnership. Although partners do not have employment rights as such, it is unlawful for a partnership to discriminate on grounds of sex, sexual orientation, disability, marital status, race, religion, ethnic origin or age when appointing a new partner, or in the way partnership benefits are shared.

The partnership is responsible for running a business, so partners will not just be involved in patient care and related administration. They will need to ensure the smooth running and development of the practice as their income depends on the annual profits. Their employees should be suitably paid and supported with appropriate modern contracts, education and training. Most high earning practices will have loyal and effective staff because the partnership has invested in them. A partnership needs a good practice manager to ensure that the partners do not have to do unnecessary management, although there will always be some management issues the partners will have to be involved with.

Profit-sharing

When deciding on a fair share of profits the partners need to look at the overall workload and this may result in a varying amount of clinical work for the same share of profit. This is one of the most difficult concepts for a new partner to grasp. Time will need to be allocated to the various activities that constitute a partner's workload. Such activities, providing the income is paid to the practice rather than the individual GP, may include hospital sessions as a clinical assistant, work as a GP with special interest (GPwSI), development of a locality service as part of the practice-based commissioning process, teaching, involvement with a PCT committee or advisory work. It may also include responsibility for on-call or out-of-hours and being the lead partner for areas such as clinical governance or IT. These are just some examples of the type of portfolio working and skills development that many GPs are becoming involved with in the course of their careers.

Some of these activities may not generate direct income for the practice, or a lesser amount than that produced from clinical work. It can be difficult to quantify in pure financial terms but benefits can be created for the practice through competent management and effective networking. For example, a GP trainer will have knowledge of new GPs that the practice may want to recruit and a partner on PCO committees will understand the impact of new initiatives for the practice.

Practices have various ways of calculating workload with some making sure everyone does a proportional share of non-clinical work and others insisting everyone does the same share of clinical work as their profit share. New partners may have a reduced share of the profits for the first 1 or 2 years while they develop additional skills. Some may feel this is unfair but many partners look back after a few years and realise that it took time before they were able to make a full contribution to the partnership.

It was described above how non-GPs can enter a partnership. Since GPs traditionally expect to earn more than nurses and managers, this may be a further reason why it is relatively rare for them to be incorporated into the partnership and profit share.

Flexibility within partnerships

Within a partnership there may be the opportunity, at various points in an individual's career, to increase or decrease workload and related share of the profits. For example, a GP who is a parent with young children may want to have a reduced workload. Similarly, an older doctor approaching retirement may wish to scale down his or her clinical or administrative commitment. However, any change can only occur with the agreement of the other partners.

Premises

Some GP partnerships own their premises and the new partner may be invited to buy a share. This will usually be offered once they have reached parity (equal profit share) and plan to stay long term in the partnership. It is important to get written confirmation that this will be an option, and under what terms, at the time of accepting a partnership. Although it may look daunting to a new partner to own premises, in most cases it is to be recommended. The partner will need a mortgage for their share but they will usually receive a compensatory rent reimbursement from their PCO, which can be offset against their mortgage payments. Any remaining mortgage costs are tax deductible and the partner will have a good investment provided the capital value of the premises increases. Buying a share of the premises should be seen as a long-term investment and independent financial advice needs to be sought before purchase.

Partnership splits

As stated above, a partnership is rather like a marriage and it is not uncommon for disputes to occur. These can be acrimonious and expensive, particularly if a watertight partnership agreement is not in place.

Contracts with PCOs

An NHS single-handed GP or partnership obtains income for NHS services via their contract with their PCO. There are four types of contract:

- The new General Medical Service contract (GMS2) was introduced in 2004 and became the standard contract for the majority of self-employed GPs, unless they chose to opt for one of the other contracts.
- Personal Medical Service (PMS) contract.
- PCO managed practice (usually a short-term arrangement during transitions between the other types of practice).
- The Alternative Provider of Medical services (APMS), which is a new development little known before 2005.

It is also possible for practices to set themselves up as limited companies, but this is currently rare.

In the United Kingdom the average full-time GP partner has a list size of 1800 patients, although this can be very variable. It is not unknown for a single-handed practices to have a list of up to 4000, though often they will employ salaried or locum doctors and nurses to share the workload.

The GMS2 practice

The GMS2 contract was introduced in April 2004. Under new arrangements contracts for medical services are now between the whole practice and the PCO rather than by individual contractors. It therefore follows that any changes in the partnership may affect the contractual relationship between the practice and the PCO.

The contract is priced via a number of mechanisms.[4] These include the number of registered patients and the Quality and Outcome Framework (QoF) points achieved. QoF points are awarded for various indicators including standards of management of chronic diseases such as diabetes. There are also additional and enhanced services the practice can choose to offer which generate additional income, such as minor surgery. As a result of the GMS2 contract there is an increasing trend for vacancies to be advertised on a salaried rather than partnership basis and this is discussed further under 'Salaried GPs'.

The PMS practice

PMS practices were introduced in 1998 to allow GPs to provide more creative services. Usually partners hold contracts as a group with their PCO but it is possible for an individual to hold a contract. PMS practices are paid from an agreed budget providing they meet targets set by their PCO. These often involve QoF points or other quality markers similar to GMS2 practice contracts. Historically PMS practices have benefited from 'growth' money to help them provide new services. In some cases they have received funding to recruit a salaried GP and free up partners time to provide other services, or to assist in introducing and providing additional services. This has continued as part of their recurrent annual budget and is one of the reasons partners in PMS practices on average earn significantly more than those in GMS2 practices.[5] However, at the time of writing, there are moves from central government are indicating a desire to move back towards more 'equal shares' and such moves may result in PMS practices loosing income.

The APMS practice

Along with traditional GP providers of general practice, APMS contracts are open to bids from commercial profit-making companies and not-for-profit organisations. These can be secondary care or community trusts or groups of GPs as well as private organisations. The NHS Improvement Plan[6] states that in the next 4 years there will be a focus on an increased choice of providers from all sectors. Already more than half of PCOs are using APMS contracts for out-of-hours services.

Setting up a new GP practice as a provider

In the current NHS model it is usually only possible to become a provider by filling a vacancy created by an existing provider retiring or resigning. PCOs will not usually agree to finance a new provider's premises, staffing or other overheads, making it financially impractical to create a profitable new practice. However, with the current sea change of the NHS structure it looks increasingly likely that sources of finance beyond the PCO (and NHS) will become available to primary care providers to create practices with a significant private investment.

Part-time partnership

In the introduction we described the drivers to changing the work/life balance for GPs and increasing numbers of GPs now wish to work as part-time partners. Many GPs have to make a choice between partnership and salaried work and the factors they must consider are described below.

Advantages of working as a partner

- Pay may be higher than for an equivalent salaried post.
- Status of running your own business.
- Control over staff appointments and management.
- Control over the way the practice runs.
- Opportunity to develop new business ideas and income streams, such as private work.
- Cannot be dismissed or made redundant (defending on the partnership agreement).
- Entitled to seniority payments.
- Certain tax advantages compared with employed status.

Disadvantages of working as a partner

- Due to the current shortage of vacancies it may be difficult to find a post in a preferred geographical locality.
- Income depends on profits, which can go up or down.
- Joint and several liability, with partners bearing partial responsibility for errors and omissions (clinical and financial).
- No minimum terms and conditions.
- Partnership agreements vary and may be difficult to negotiate (especially if wanting to work flexibly).
- If there is a workforce shortfall the partners have responsibility to meet the need irrespective of their partnership contract.
- Potentially unlimited workload, which is dependent on patient demand.
- May be difficult to ensure the workload is split fairly according to profit share.
- If a part-time GP has a low superannuable income no seniority payment is payable, although there are certain protections for GPs in low earning practices.

- Some partnerships will divide payments for work such as appraisal according to profit share, despite the time required to do the work being equal for all partners.
- Maternity locum cover payments from the PCO will not cover the actual cost of the maternity leave.
- Need to purchase own locum insurance to cover for any sick leave.
- High medical protection costs.
- If a partnership dispute leads to a split the partners are responsible for managing the fall-out.
- Employees can take the partners to a tribunal or sue for grievances.
- Responsible for the performance of employed staff.
- Responsible for health and safety at work.
- May be responsible for the maintenance of the practice premises.

Clearly a partnership is a big undertaking and any GP considering this is advised to seek professional advice at an early stage.

Salaried GPs

Definition

A salaried GP has a contract of employment with a practice, PCO or APMS to provide GP services for a defined number of hours per week. The term 'salaried' GP should be distinguished from 'sessional' GP, the latter being an umbrella term to include all GPs who are not partners in a practice, including locums. Locums are self-employed and work on a freelance basis. All sessional GPs are 'performers' in that they must be accepted on the performer list of a PCO before they are eligible to work as an NHS GP.

Salaried GPs include a variety of post titles including assistant, PMS salaried GP, retainer and returner. Historically anyone not wanting to take up a partnership worked as an assistant, often with rather poor pay and benefits. In many cases they were women working part-time for what was perceived as 'pin-money'. In recent years organisations such as the General Practitioner Committee and National Association of Sessional GPs have lobbied for better rights for salaried GPs.

Benefits of salaried work

Salaried posts appeal to GPs for many different reasons. GPs who have just completed training or who have heavy domestic responsibilities often don't want the burden of partnership, preferring to concentrate on clinical work. Some new GPs also lack the confidence to manage their own business, feeling unprepared at this stage in their career. For GPs with spouses or partners who are likely to move around the country (such as junior doctors) a partnership may not be a realistic commitment. GPs undertaking portfolio careers, with significant workload in areas such as research, education or management, may find a salaried post allows them to maintain their clinical interest and skills in controlled hours, leaving time and energy for their other work. For GPs nearing retirement, a salaried post may be a way of reducing workload while maintaining their role of caring for their patients.

The relatively high availability of salaried posts compared with partnerships since 2005 is probably primarily due to the widening gap between partnership and salaried income that has occurred under GMS2. In addition, under the previous GMS arrangements, the basic practice allowance was paid to individual practitioners and hence was part of the practice income, so when a partner left a practice the practice would lose that income. Under GMS2 because the contract for GMS is between the practice and the PCO and there are no individual registered patient lists the basic practice allowance ceased to exist. Practices are able to be creative with their posts and choose whether to replace or newly appoint a partner with a salaried GP or an alternative practitioner.

Salaried contracts

The BMA has produced model contracts for the main types of salaried posts[7–9] but PMS and APMS posts are not included because they are 'independent'. The model contracts contain clearly stated benefits such as sick leave and a defined job plan to clarify hours worked and duties undertaken, in line with the terms and conditions of other salaried doctors in the NHS. The National Health Service (General Medical Services Contracts) Regulations 2004 (Statutory Instrument 2004, number 291) states: 'The contractor shall only offer employment to a general medical practitioner on terms and conditions which are no less favourable than those contained in the Model terms and conditions of service for a salaried general practitioner employed by a GMS practice.' Unfortunately not all practices and PCOs choose to follow this guidance and it is up to the individual doctors to ensure they have a good quality contract, which is implemented.

In theory it is possible to have a temporary salaried contract as a GP. However, recent changes to employment law mean that after 2 years of continuous employment the right to continue (unless made redundant) is acquired.

Although employing a salaried GP may initially appear more cost-effective for the practice than engaging a new partner, the quality of the terms and conditions of employment within the new GMS2 salaried GP model contract has resulted (in some cases) in a narrowing of the cost gap between a salaried

GP and partner. In addition the tax rules in this country make the gross cost of a salaried GP greater than a partner for the same net income.

One of the outcomes of the salaried model contract is that a job plan should be agreed upon and that the salaried GP cannot be expected to perform an unlimited amount of work. Consequently, if there is an increase in workload and/or shortfall in manpower it will be for the partners to deal with this, without resuming an increase in workload for the salaried GP.

Doctors employed by APMS organisations need to remember that there is no model contract for APMS workers and the organisation does not have to become a recognised NHS employing authority or a member of the NHS superannuation scheme. Without NHS employment, continuity of service for maternity or sickness may be lost and time employed does not count towards NHS seniority. There are no minimum terms and conditions of employment and maternity leave may be less beneficial than those of the NHS Scheme. Therefore any GP planning to work for an APMS provider needs to seek individual advice from the BMA on the contract offered, as well as thinking carefully about the long-term implications for such a post on their NHS pension and benefits such as maternity leave, paternity leave, sick leave and continuity of service.

Flexibility of salaried work

Salaried general practice is possibly the most flexible career choice in medicine (except freelance work). Providing an accommodating employer can be found it is possible for a salaried GP to work as little as 3–4 hours a week and not necessarily even in one sitting. Therefore sessions can often be fitted into school hours. Out-of-hours work for a co-op can be undertaken exclusively at nights or weekends, which would be an excellent option for a GP with children hoping to manage without childcare by dovetailing their hours with a spouse or partner working a standard 9–5 day. However, a note of caution must be given for a GP working very short hours or only for a co-op. In order to maintain professional skills many GP educators believe a minimum of two to three sessions of patient contact per week is needed. Feedback from referrals made, tests ordered and seeing patients who return for follow-up or seeking further advice is of great benefit for continuing professional development (CPD). Doctors working exclusively for co-ops or as freelance GPs may lack such feedback with the risk of becoming deskilled. They may also lack opportunities to discuss difficult cases with colleagues, participate in audit and interact with a multidisciplinary team, all of which can enhance professional development. As a result they may have difficulty providing high quality evidence of learning and development achievements at their appraisal. These issues will have to be addressed in arrangements for revalidation.

Advantages of salaried work compared with partnership

A number of areas on the list below are dependent on the type of contract, which should be carefully checked by an employment expert before accepting a post.

- Relatively larger number of posts available to choose from.
- Income is not dependent on profits.
- No joint and several liability (provided the non-partner status is defined on practice documents such as headed paper).
- Minimum terms and conditions of employment in GMS and PCO posts.
- Paid CPD (with a model contract) and (in some cases) mentoring/supervision within the practice.
- If there is a workforce shortfall or grievance it is probably not the responsibility of the salaried GP.
- Defined workload (assuming a model contract with job plan).
- Someone else (a partner) takes the overall responsibility for the practice and is there as a fallback to help with difficult clinical cases.
- Paid sick, compassionate, adoptive and maternity leave.
- Lower medical protection costs.
- No need to purchase locum insurance.
- No need to purchase property.
- Leaving the practice is less complex than if a partnership agreement were involved.

Disadvantages of salaried work compared with partnership

- Pay may be lower than an equivalent partnership post.
- Do not have the status of running a business.
- No control over staff appointments or management.
- No control over the way the practice runs.
- May not have opportunity to pursue areas of interest such a minor surgery if practice decides against offering such a service.
- Limited opportunity to develop new business ideas and income streams such as private work.
- Can be dismissed or made redundant.
- May be hard to persuade a practice to fully implement the contract, including CPD time and payments for appraisal.
- Not entitled to seniority payments.
- Employed status means fewer tax allowances.

- General practice is still rooted in the concept that partners are committed and other GPs are less committed (lower status).
- Not always possible to receive payment for their contribution to the practice's achievement under the Quality and Outcomes Framework (QoF).
- Part-time GPs need the same education as full-time GPs, but are usually allocated less protected CPD time.
- Attending practice meetings is an important part of the job; do part-time GPs attend on their day off?
- Sessional GPs are under represented on local medical committees (LMCs).

Threat to the salaried role from other practitioners

Practices are increasingly using nurse practitioners to take on the more routine aspects of a GP's role. This is probably resulting in fewer salaried posts being advertised than in the past. Physician's assistants are a type of practitioner originating from the USA now being trained to work in NHS settings such as primary care. Their role will inevitably overlap with that of the GP and this is being promoted by the current (labour) Government. These practitioners generally have lower salaries than that expected by a salaried GP, reflecting their shorter and less intense training. However, studies looking at cost-effectiveness of nurse practitioners have failed to demonstrate an advantage over salaried GPs, in part because they tend to work more slowly with longer appointment slots.[10] A debate is ongoing as to whether such practitioners are as good as fully trained GPs at decision-making under pressure, dealing with uncertainty and managing complex cases. Many questions remain as to whether such practitioners can effectively take over the whole of a salaried GP's role.

Summary

Never before has there been such a wide range of permanent posts available to GPs but partnerships are increasingly hard to come by. There are many benefits to salaried work, in particular with a BMA model contract giving protection to hours worked and employment rights. However, this model contract is often not used by PMS practices and is unlikely to be offered by APMS providers (along with an NHS pension). Salaried GPs need to ensure they are offered pay and conditions commensurate with their experience and expertise.

Over the past few years there has been an increase in the number of part-time salaried posts available, particularly in comparison with partnership. For many GPs, especially those with heavy domestic responsibilities, this career path allows the maintenance of clinical skills and enjoyment of patient contact without the burden of partnership responsibility. More recently non-medical practitioners have begun to take over parts of the traditional role of the GP and may in future threaten the position of salaried GPs, if they prove to be more cost-effective. The many benefits of partnership are not to be underestimated and it remains an attractive option for those happy to take on the burden of running their own practice and looking for long-term job security as well as continuity of patient care.

References

1 Jones L, Fisher T (2006) Workforce trends in general practice in the UK. *British Journal General Practice* **56**:124–136.
2 http://www.dh.gov.uk/PolicyAndGuidance/HumanResourcesAndTraining/Model Employer/ImprovingWorkingLives/fs/en
3 http://www.hmrc.gov.uk/manuals/bimmanual/BIM72505.htm
4 Department of Health (2004) *GMS Statement of Financial Entitlements for 2004/5.* London: Department of Health. www.dh.gov.uk/assetRoot/04/06/71/92/04067192.pdf.
5 Information Centre for Health and Social Care. *UK GP Earnings 2004/2005.* http://www.ic.nhs.uk/pubs/gpearnex0405
6 Department of Health (2004) *The NHS Improvement Plan.* Department of Health: London. http://www.bjhc.co.uk/autumnforum/docs/NHS%20Improvement%20plan.pdf
7 British Medical Association (2003) *Model Terms and Conditions of Service for a Salaried General Practitioner Employed by a GMS Practice.* London: BMA.
8 British Medical Association (2003) *Model Terms and Conditions of Service for a Salaried General Practitioner Employed by a Primary Care Trust (PCT).* London: BMA.
9 British Medical Association (2005) *Model GP Retainer Scheme Contract.* London: BMA.
10 http://www.rcgp.org.uk/pdf/ISS

Further information

1. BMA; the general practitioners committee has a sessional GP bulletin. www.bma.org.uk
2. NASGP (National Association of Sessional GPs, previously NANP). Visit their website and join this national association, they have a myriad of information about the various types of working. www.nasgp.org.uk
3. Doctors' Support Line: telephone 0870 765 0001; www.doctorssupport.org
4. Medical Women's Federation www.medicalwomensfederation.co.uk: an independent charity which supports the professional development of women in medicine.

Chapter 12 **Portfolio working**

Maria Elliott

Introduction

So, you would like to be a general practitioner (GP), but not one who works 10 sessions a week in face-to-face contact with patients for the next 40 years. Few people would choose to do that nowadays. Modern general practice offers unprecedented opportunities for a portfolio career.

A *portfolio* is a collection of works representing a person's ability and achievement within his or her particular field. The concept of the portfolio has long been established in the media and art world. More recently education, including medical education, has adopted the principles of the portfolio.[1,2] Long gone are the days of the single-handed GP practising from his own home with his wife as his receptionist and/or nurse. Most of his time would have been spent on consulting in his surgery and visiting patients at home. GPs nowadays practice from purpose built premises, often as a member of a large primary healthcare team (PHCT).

Portfolio career

Following their undergraduate studies and final examinations, young doctors enter the Foundation School programme which lasts 2 years. Those that choose general practice will complete another 3 years of vocational training the last of which is spent in general practice, under the guidance of a GP trainer. On satisfactory completion of the 3-year programme and passing the new MRCGP examination the doctor will be awarded the Certificate of Completion of Training. From then on she or he is able to practise independently as a general practitioner. I have been a GP trainer for the last 23 years and during that time have trained 21 registrars. For the first 18 years or

Choosing General Practice: Your Career Guide. Edited by Anne Hastie and Anne Stephenson. © 2008 Blackwell Publishing, ISBN: 978-1-4501-7070-3.

so, most of my registrars entered partnerships as soon as they finished their vocational training and spent all or most of the working week consulting in their surgeries. Latterly there has been a sea change in young GPs' attitudes to working in general practice. Few of them want to settle straight away into partnerships; most of them wish to continue with some sessional GP scheme with an educational component.

Innovative GP posts have mushroomed, often under the aegis of Academic Departments of General Practice and Primary Care Trusts (PCTs). These posts combine clinical sessions in general practice and part-time training in hospitals or the community in a chosen specialty, often leading to a diploma or MSc. The GP may subsequently specialise in that subject and work as a GPwSI (GP with Specialist Interest). Some of the innovative posts offer opportunities for research or teaching.

Locum work allows young doctors to experience general practice in different settings including comparing and contrasting the working environment of urban and rural practices. Many doctors choose to work abroad for a period of time before settling into partnerships.

Working as a partner or salaried doctor in general practice offers stability and, eventually, most qualified GPs will settle for this option. Working as a member of the PHCT hugely increases one's job satisfaction. The vast majority of doctors entering general practice do not want to work full-time in the practice. There is a huge number of special interests that GPs can pursue and they divide their working week to suit these. Over the years, GPs can move from one interest to another, reinvigorating their careers and stopping burnout. Few hospital specialists are afforded this luxury. I will highlight some of the choices open to GPs as part of their portfolio working. The following is a non-exhaustive list of possible career options:

• *GpwSI:* in a variety of specialties working either in a hospital on a sessional basis or within the general practice taking referrals from neighbouring practices. This will be one of the key elements of practice-based commissioning, resulting in fewer referrals to hospitals. Some of the specialties that GPs in our PCT have taken on so far are dermatology, rheumatology, diabetes, substance misuse, urology, family planning, palliative care, sports medicine, refugee health and working with the homeless.

• *Working in service development and management:* either within the practice, PCT or on a national level. GPs are increasingly taking a lead role in this area. Various management courses on offer enable GPs to get skilled in this work.

• *Teaching in general practice* has been the most rewarding and enjoyable part of my working life. There is scope to get involved in undergraduate and postgraduate medical education, teaching allied health professionals or health education in schools just to name a few. Increasing numbers of GPs undertake educational courses to facilitate their teaching and some achieve a diploma or master's degree in medical education.

• *Academic posts in general practice departments* are often part-time, enabling the doctors to continue with their clinical work, whilst pursuing academic interests in education or research.

• *Medical politics* play an important role in the future development of general practice. The Local Medical Committee members are elected from local GPs and some GPs will serve on national bodies such as the General Practice Committee, General Medical Council or British Medical Association.

• *Working as a police surgeon or prison doctor* is another area of specialism GPs can engage in.

• *Occupational heath* looks after people in their working environment and GPs can play an important role in health and safety at work.

• *Medical journalism* combines an individual's creative literary skill with clinical work.

Summary

In our time, when medical science develops with unprecedented speed and doctors face constant changes in their work, one of the greatest challenges for young GPs is how to stop burnout. Working full-time in the same surgery throughout one's working life no longer seems an acceptable working pattern for most GPs. A portfolio career enables GPs to reinvigorate themselves periodically with a new interest, inject fresh enthusiasm into their working life and prolong their professional career.

References

1 Thistlethwaite J (2006) How to keep a portfolio. *The Clinical Teacher* 3(2): 118–123.
2 Pearson DJ, Heywood P (2004) Portfolio use in general practice vocational training: a survey of GP registrars. *Medical Education* **38**: 87–95.

Chapter 13 **Academic general practice**

Anne Stephenson, Neil Jackson and Roger Jones

Introduction

The development of academic general practice

Academic general practice forms part of clinical academic medicine. Clinical academics are doctors who combine their clinical work with a variable proportion of academic work – research and teaching. Academic general practice is located in universities and medical schools, with every UK medical school now having at least one professor of general practice or primary care, and also in the postgraduate deaneries, which have responsibilities for postgraduate training and contribute significantly to the career development of academic general practitioners.

The foundations of academic general practice were laid in the nineteenth century, by James MacKenzie and William Pickles (see Box 13.1), whose pioneering studies in cardiology, infectious diseases and epidemiology were carried out years ahead of their time. Patrick Byrne and John Hunt were instrumental in establishing the College, later the Royal College of General Practitioners, in the 1950s and 1960s, and the College has played a significant role in supporting academic general practice every since.

The father of research in general practice in the United Kingdom in more recent years was John Fry, a single-handed general practitioner working in Beckenham, Kent, whose detailed recordings of all his patient contacts over an extended period provided the first descriptions of the workload of general practice and the natural history of the common minor and major illnesses encountered by GPs, as summarised in his landmark publication *Common Diseases*[1] and numerous other publications.

The first professor of general practice, Richard Scott, was appointed in Edinburgh in 1963, and over the next decade academic general practitioners

---

Choosing General Practice: Your Career Guide. Edited by Anne Hastie and Anne Stephenson. © 2008 Blackwell Publishing, ISBN: 978-1-4501-7070-3.

Box 13.1 Early UK general practice academics

Sir James MacKenzie, a Scottish general practitioner (GP) born in 1853 and Fellow of the Royal Society, had over 50 papers published, mainly in cardiology, as well as setting up a research institute in St Andrews and running a very busy practice.

William Pickles, born in Leeds in 1885, was a country GP and famous epidemiologist. He published a medical classic in 1939, *Epidemiology in Country Practice*, that described his observations. He was the first President of the College of General Practitioners.

Patrick Byrne, born in Birkenhead near Liverpool in 1913, was the first to run teacher training courses for GPs, published a very influential book on communication between doctors and patients (*Doctors Talking with Patients*), was the a founder member of the College of General Practitioners in 1952 (to become the Royal College of General Practitioners, RCGP, in 1967), became Professor of General Practice in Manchester in 1972 and was President of the RCGP 1973–6.

John Hunt, born in India in 1905, was a GP in London, helped set up the College of General Practitioners (being its first Honorary Secretary from 1953 to 1966 and its President from 1967 to 1970) and was instrumental in the raising of standards and development of general practice in the United Kingdom.

John Fry, born in Croydon in 1922, was a general practitioner in Kent who meticulously recorded every consultation that took place in his practice for 40 years; described, analysed and published his findings and as a result became a highly respected and influential researcher.

laid the foundations for the evidence base which would inform clinical work in general practice for years ahead. John Howie in Edinburgh built on the descriptive work of Fry, and brought experimental method to research in general practice. David Metcalfe in Manchester and John Bain in Aberdeen and Southampton were among the first to study the patient–doctor interaction in the consultation in detail, and others such as Paul Freeling in London conducted studies into the interactions between physical and psychological disorders in primary care. David Morrell, also working in London, was among the first to study the reasons for patients' consultation with minor illness and the ways in which common medical problems could best be managed in general practice and by patients themselves. The driving force behind their research, and much of what followed, was the recognition of the need to equip general practice with its own research evidence to guide diagnosis and management, rather than relying on observations and studies conducted in hospital settings.

Academic general practice organisations

The Association of University Teachers in General Practice had its first scientific meeting in Cardiff in 1972, and the name reflected the fact that teaching was the principal function of academic general practitioners at that time. As research activity in the university departments grew, the name of the organisation was changed to the Association of University Departments of General Practice (AUDGP) in 1992, and the annual scientific meetings of the AUDGP became the focus for the presentation of the original research work undertaken by academic GPs. The AUDGP was, in turn, re-christened the Society for Academic Primary Care (SAPC), in part in recognition of the growing importance of non-clinical researchers – medical sociologists, psychologists, nurses, epidemiologists and others – in the conduct of increasingly complex research studies in primary care. The SAPC is now the national organisation in the United Kingdom which not only hosts the annual scientific meeting for academic general practice but has also acted as a political and lobbying organisation, seeking to improve funding for teaching and research in general practice and to establish career structures for clinical and non-clinical academics working in primary care.

Postgraduate deaneries

The postgraduate deaneries have, in the past, been regarded as principally NHS rather than academic organisations, although many if not all have well-established relationships with local universities whilst being an integral part of the Strategic Health Authorities in England (arrangements for deaneries in the other three UK countries and for the Tri-Services/Defence deanery vary according to the structure and administration of the relevant healthcare system). The traditional deanery role has encompassed the commissioning, management and quality assurance of postgraduate medical education and training. However, since the establishment of the Postgraduate Medical Education and Training Board (PMETB) in 2005 as a statutory body it has assumed the role of assuring the quality control processes of deaneries. Postgraduate departments of general practice within deaneries have also had a traditional provider function where part-time departmental medical and non-medical staff and educators employed in the wider educational network have been actively involved in teaching and the provision of courses and educational programmes for GP trainees, new GPs and established GPs. The education provider role has also extended into the wider development of the multiprofessional/multidisciplinary primary care workforce. There are also opportunities for international work to support the development of family medicine and primary care in overseas healthcare systems. Postgraduate GP departments have also expanded their academic activities to include presentations at national and international conferences, writing and publishing books and peer-reviewed papers, usually with reference to the growing speciality of medical education or NHS workforce issues.

Working as an academic GP

Teaching
The principal responsibilities of a university department of general practice and primary care are to provide a programme of education for undergraduate medical students in general practice and community settings, to conduct research studies in general practice and primary care, and to publish their results in peer-reviewed journals. General practice teaching extends across all years of the undergraduate curriculum and nationally contributes to between 10 and 15% of curriculum time. These large and complex teaching programmes, which are mostly funded by Service Increment for Teaching (SIFT) in England and Wales and the Additional Costs of Teaching (ACT) funding in Scotland, are delivered by academic GPs with particular teaching responsibilities, working closely with teaching administrators and co-ordinators, and large numbers of NHS GPs who act as community-based GP tutors.

Research
Research in general practice is now big business, and most successful university departments have annual research grant incomes running into the millions of pounds, and general practice research is published widely in primary care journals such as the *British Journal of General Practice* and *Family Practice,* in general medical journals such as the *BMJ* and *Lancet* and also in specialist journals, depending on the subject of the research. Most departments concentrate on particular research themes, and try to sustain long-term programmes of research in particular areas, although because of the generalist nature of primary care and the highly competitive funding environment in which research operates, an opportunistic approach to research grant acquisition is also required.

A typical university department is likely to be led by one or more professors of general practice, with other senior academic staff (professors, readers and senior lecturers) representing a range of other disciplines, such as medical sociology and clinical epidemiology. There are likely to be a number of lecturers and some research training fellows, with larger numbers of research associates and research assistants working on specific projects, all supported by administrative and secretarial staff. Many of these posts will be permanent appointments, with core funding from the university and sometimes the NHS, with other staff working on short-term contracts, generally research grants and research training posts of a fixed duration.

Working in a university department

Academic general practice provides a stimulating and satisfying career. Whilst maintaining patient contact, either in a practice co-located with the university department, or, more typically, in a practice in another part of town, the academic GP has protected time for research and teaching. In the early phases of an academic career, described in more detail later, research fellows and lecturers will need to 'learn the trade' by getting involved in both teaching and research. A specified research project is likely to be the basis for a research training fellowship at both pre-doctoral and post-doctoral stages, but in order to put together a curriculum vitae for further job applications experience and skills in both teaching and research are going to be needed. With increasing seniority the amount of clinical work is likely to reduce, and broader research, teaching and administrative responsibilities will enter the picture. Variety is always likely to be the key ingredient, and almost certainly provides protection from some of the more repetitive aspects of service practice, whilst at the same time offering opportunity to have a real impact on medical students' lives and to see the fruits of your research in print. Balancing all of these aspects of an academic life can be challenging, but is ultimately extremely rewarding.

It has to be said, however, that the attractiveness of clinical academic medicine has varied over the years, and at present, partly because of salary differentials, recruitment rates across all clinical academic disciplines are relatively low. It is likely that as the recommendations of the Walport Report,[2] discussed later, are implemented, the situation will improve, and it is important to remember that whilst basic salaries in clinical academic medicine do not compare favourably with higher-earning NHS practices, clinical academic GPs are, like all other consultants, eligible for Clinical Excellence Awards which, with increasing seniority, represent a substantial enhancement of academic salary scales.

Getting started

Modern undergraduate medical curricula emphasise the importance of research in a doctor's development and professional life and evidence-based medicine is seen as essential in the content of knowledge and skills teaching (see below). The inclusion of the student voice in the evaluation of teaching is also widespread and optional modules and intercalated BSc degrees in medical education are now being introduced into undergraduate medical curricula. Before long all medical students will be expected to have had some training and experience in teaching as well as research and will be further trained in both areas throughout their early postgraduate and specialty training years. With intense competition to get good training posts and consultant jobs, more and more young doctors are doing research and obtaining MDs and PhDs as well as being trained and involved in teaching, developing their teaching portfolios. A decision to enter academic general practice can be made as an undergraduate or it can be entered at any stage along your training path and career. It is probably best to start early if you want to become an established academic but some GPs 'get the bug' later in their careers and it is never too late to start. Some view academic general practice as their primary career and others as a special interest in their normal work as a general practitioner. The curiosity and determination to find out how something works or might work and the passion to communicate one's knowledge and experience to others is a strong antidote to boredom, antipathy and burnout.

Postgraduate academic teaching in general practice

The GP trainer may be regarded as proficient or an expert in general practice, exhibiting the features of personal mastery.[3] Although the influence of the GP trainer as a role model for the GP registrar is often profound, the very essence of the trainer/trainee relationship is the dynamic two-way educational process whereby the GP trainer can also learn from the GP registrar. This is particularly so when the registrar comes into the training practice fresh from the secondary care part of the training equipped with the knowledge of the latest advances in hospital medicine.

The attributes or characteristics of the GP trainer are many and may be classified under three main headings:

- *The trainer as a doctor:* appropriate knowledge, skills and attitudes as a clinician
- *The trainer as a teacher:* personal qualities, preparation for lecturing, organisation of teaching, teaching abilities, use of assessment methodology
- *The training practice:* premises, staffing, record systems, library facilities/ teaching aids, etc.

In terms of personal mastery and academic teaching the GP trainer must exhibit these attributes and demonstrate the required quality standards and it is hoped that the GP registrar as the apprentice will aspire to achieve these high levels of practice during the time spent in the training environment.

Teaching styles

Teaching styles have previously been defined in *The Future General Practitioner: Learning and Teaching.*[4] Here the authors emphasise that the teacher (or 'master') must have an awareness of what his or her trainee (or 'apprentice') needs to learn. Inherent to this is the competence of the teacher to help the trainee in identifying what is required to be learned and to stimulate the process of appropriate self-directed learning. The authors go on to identify four teaching styles which maybe exhibited by the GP trainer.

- *Authoritarian – To 'tell and sell'*: A domineering approach where facts are passed from trainer to trainee. Here the teacher may not encourage questioning by the trainee which could challenge his or her authority or 'mastership'.
- *Socratic – 'Teaching by question and answer'*: The teacher always asks and the trainee always answers. This in turn acts as a trigger for more questions and the teacher imparts new facts when the trainee (as the learner) demonstrates areas of deficiency or ignorance.
- *Heuristic – 'To find out for yourself'*: Encouraging the trainee to take responsibility for self-directed learning – that is to say 'learning by doing'.
- *Counselling:* A less directive style with the aim of encouraging the trainee to understand the interactions taking place between him/herself and the material being learned.

The GP trainer

The ideal GP trainer should be an exponent of these different styles, which can be applied in a range of different situations. In practice, however, all GP trainers have strengths and weaknesses as teachers and therefore this may not be possible. The accomplished GP trainer will be aware of his or her weaknesses and will compensate for these by other means to the advantage of the trainee. More about the role and responsibilities of teachers in undergraduate and postgraduate general practice can be found in the chapter on teaching in general practice.

Evidence-based medicine and work-based learning

There are various definitions of evidence-based medicine (EBM). Sacket et al. (1996) describe EBM as 'the conscientious, explicit and judicious use of current best evidence in making decisions about the care of individual patients. The practice of evidence-based medicine means integrating individual clinical expertise with the best available clinical evidence from systematic research.'[5]

Various definitions of work-based learning (WBL) exist. Barr has defined WBL as 'work located' or 'work related'; i.e. it takes place at work or away from work with the objective of improving work performance.[6] Seagraves and colleagues define WBL as learning which takes place at, from or for work.[7] In this definition 'at' relates to the place where learning occurs, 'from' relates

> **Box 13.2** The benefits of work-based learning (WBL) in the new NHS
>
> • WBL enables a collaborative approach between institutes of higher education, employers and employees, to the ultimate benefit of patients using the NHS.
> • WBL promotes formal and informal collaborative learning at practice level.
> • Learning which takes place at work can be given academic recognition while taking into account both present and future roles of employees.
> • WBL can promote both individual and team development within NHS organisations.
> • WBL should enable a balance to be achieved between personal fulfilment for individual healthcare professionals and the wider needs for the employing organisation and the NHS as a whole.
> • WBL allows a flexible approach to the timing, location and methods of learning.
> • WBL promotes self-motivation, critical thinking and reflective practice.
> • WBL enhances a greater understanding of working within the complex environment of the new NHS.

to the stimulus that promotes learning, and 'for' represents the purpose of learning.

WBL can be used to promote higher standards of patient care by looking primarily at the requirements of patients, as it is their problems that are central to the considerations of any new or developing healthcare service. It could also encourage all professional groups to seek to provide the correct patient pathways through the development of joint learning and the improvement of inter-professional relationships. Not only is it beneficial to improve communications between professionals at all levels, but it is also important to redefine roles to maximise efficiency in all aspects of care distribution.

Burton and Jackson have previously described the benefits of WBL in the new NHS in the United Kingdom (see Box 13.2).[8]

WBL as a model of lifelong learning can enable healthcare professionals working as individuals and in teams in the NHS to participate in regular and systematic educational and research activity. By ensuring that the application of principles of EBM is firmly embedded in a system of WBL, this in turn will contribute to the maintenance and development of clinical competence and performance, while promoting critical thinking, reflective practice and quality care for patients. A firm partnership between WBL and EBM in general practice will also ensure that lifelong learning for all healthcare professionals is appropriate to meet the challenges of a fast-changing world, medical advances, new technologies and new approaches to patient care.

Training to become an academic general practitioner

The Walport Report of 2005,[2] in response to a perceived lack of career structure, flexibility and support for clinical medical careers, made recommendations which have led to a number of initiatives.

1 The provision of more intercalated BSc degrees during undergraduate medical training.
2 Increased opportunities for medical students to learn about the theory and practice of medical education.
3 MD-PhD Schemes for new graduates.
4 Academic foundation programmes.
5 Dedicated academic training programmes during specialist training.
6 A variety of entry points into and out of academic training programmes.
7 Creation of a cohort of new senior lectureship posts funded in partnership between the NHS Trusts, Universities Departments of Health and other research funders.
8 Pay parity of clinical academics with NHS counterparts.

In addition recommendations were made for academic GPs with the creation of 4-year training posts of which 2 years would be academic including, for example, a Master's degree, as well as special 1-year funding opportunities for GPs who have completed a PhD and who need to prepare an application for a postdoctoral fellowship. Rates of pay for senior academic GPs were also increased to be commensurate with those of other senior clinical academics. As a result of these recommendations and the start of their implementation, academic medicine is becoming a more attractive and better supported proposition. It is important to get a good basic training in research and/or teaching if you want to embark on an academic career and at present there are a number of entry points that you might consider.

Academic foundation posts

As in 2007, 5% of Year 2 Foundation posts, funded centrally, are dedicated to academic medicine, either as a dedicated 4-month post or as an integrated academic programme throughout the second foundation year. Four-month foundation posts in general practice occur in the second foundation year and of these, at present, six are academic. This would be a good introduction to academic medicine early in your career and if you were interested you could talk with deaneries and departments about the possibilities.

Academic registrar posts

Academic registrar posts are now available through many deaneries. They are generally a part of 4-year programmes of GP training, i.e. 3 years of specialist

GP training with an additional 1 year of academic training generally integrated into the last 18 months or 2 years of the programme.

Master's degree in primary care

Many University Departments of General Practice offer master's degrees in primary care. These can be taken by GPs at any stage and are often also open to other members of the primary healthcare team. Many Primary Care Trust schemes allow GPs to do this either part-time over 2 years or as a full-time 1-year sabbatical. Most GPs choose to do the part-time option. An MSc consists of a formal taught element in research skills and often educational theory and practice as well as the requirement to complete a research project and produce a dissertation. Part-time MScs usually require students to spend 1 day a week at the department and 1 day a week doing self-directed study such as reading essay writing and project work.

Fellowships for an MD or a PhD

These are for GPs who have had some training in and experience of research. Such a fellowship and degree would be an important step in becoming a senior academic. Many research bodies offer fellowships and if this is what you are interested in it is worth talking with your local or favoured Department of General Practice. Fellowships are also advertised in journals such as the *British Medical Journal* or the *British Journal of General Practice*. You will need a connection to an academic department to do this and successful candidates would generally get 3 years of funding to complete the degree. You would also be expected to publish your findings in a peer-reviewed journal.

Teacher training courses and qualifications

For new teachers there are usually a number of introductory courses available either through your local deanery for postgraduate teaching or through your Department of General Practice for undergraduate teaching. Deaneries and universities are increasingly working together to run teacher training courses as much of the knowledge and skills are transferable. Universities also have generic certificates, diplomas and degrees in education which are worth exploring and there are degrees in medical education available that you can find if you look on the internet. Once again it is well worth seeking advice and support from your local Department of General Practice or Deanery.

A sabbatical

If you are a hard working GP why not consider taking a sabbatical to pursue an academic training and undertake research or teaching? It is a very good way to take a break from clinical commitments while at the same time learning some new skills that will benefit your career and the health and care of patients. You would need to talk with your practice and with your Primary Care Trust about such plans and give yourself plenty of time to do so. Some imaginative practices include funding for sabbaticals as part of their overall business planning.

With the recent focus on encouraging doctors to enter academia there will be new initiatives that we have not listed here and the best way to find out about these is to contact your local Deanery or Department of General Practice.

Portfolio career approach

For most GPs academic medicine is part of their portfolio of activities (see more in Chapter 12). This is a reflection of the way in which doctors who work in general practice has changed over time in relation to flexible working patterns in primary care and the wider NHS. This has particular importance in view of the increase in the feminisation of the GP workforce in recent years. A portfolio career approach can enhance job satisfaction and allow other individual life priorities to be fitted into the working week which typically might include service provision sessions in a practice, undergraduate teaching, studying for a higher degree, research activity, writing a book, etc. Portfolio careers in general practice also bring benefits to the wider NHS as well as individual practitioners by promoting recruitment and retention in the GP workforce.

Conclusion

In the new NHS the enhancement of academic general practice remains a priority for the future to meet the challenges of a fast-changing world, medical advances, new technologies and new approaches to patient care. At an individual level academic medicine enlivens and supports a career in general practice. In the United Kingdom most academic general practitioners are either working in academic university departments as researchers and/or teachers, or have strong links to postgraduate deaneries where they participate in continuing professional development programmes.

Useful contacts

Society for Academic Primary Care website.
    http://www.sapc.ac.uk/
Deanery finder website.
    http://www.gprecruitment.org.uk/deanery/map.htm

Association for the Study of Medical Education website.
http://www.asme.org.uk/
Modernising Medical Careers website.
http://www.mmc.nhs.uk/pages/home

References

1 Fry J (1979) *Common Diseases: Their Nature, Incidence and Care.* Lancaster: MTP Press.
2 Modernising Medical Careers. Medically and dentally qualified academic staff: recommendations for training the researchers and educators of the future. *Report of the Academic Careers Sub-Committee of Modernising Medical Careers and the UK Clinical Research Collaboration.* http://www.mmc.nhs.uk/download_files/Medically-and-Dentally-Qualified-academic-staff-recommendations-Report.pdf (accessed 30 April 2007)
3 Souster V, Jackson N (2003) Apprenticeship systems and work based learning. In: Burton J, Jackson N (eds) *Work Based Learning in Primary Care.* Oxford: Radcliffe.
4 Royal College of General Practitioners (1972) *The Future General Practitioner: Learning and Teaching.* London: RCGP.
5 Sacket DL, Rosenberg WM, Gray JA, Haynes RB, Richardson WS (1996) Evidence based medicine: what it is and what it isn't. *British Medical Journal* **312**: 71–72.
6 Barr H (2003) Interprofessional issues and work based learning. In: Burton J, Jackson N (eds) *Work Based Learning in Primary Care.* Oxford: Radcliffe.
7 Seagraves L, Osborne N, Neal P, et al. (1996) *Learning in Smaller Companies: Final Report.* Stirling: University of Stirling.
8 Burton J, Jackson N (2003) Theory and practice of work based learning in the new NHS. In: Burton J, Jackson N (eds) *Work Based Learning in Primary Care.* Oxford: Radcliffe.

Chapter 14 **Teaching in general practice**

Amanda Platts and Anne Stephenson

Why teach? And why teach in general practice?

Those working in general practice have always earned more from their seeing patients than in teaching, whether it be undergraduate teaching or postgraduate teaching. Why do so many enthusiastic general practitioners (GPs) still become trainers of GP specialist registrars, support medical students and run courses? What is the big attraction of teaching?

Societal expectations and professional responsibility

The General Medical Council (GMC) lists the responsibilities of good medical practice for all doctors[1] and this includes a section (paragraphs 15–19) on teaching and training, appraising and assessing.

- Teaching, training, appraising and assessing doctors and students are important for the care of patients now and in the future. You should be willing to contribute to these activities.
- If you are involved in teaching you must develop the skills, attitudes and practices of a competent teacher.
- You must make sure that all staff for whom you are responsible, including locums and students, are properly supervised.
- You must be honest and objective when appraising or assessing the performance of colleagues, including locums and students. Patients will be put at risk if you describe as competent someone who has not reached or maintained a satisfactory standard of practice.
- You must provide only honest, justifiable and accurate comments when giving references for, or writing reports about, colleagues. When providing references you must do so promptly and include all information that is relevant to your colleague.

Choosing General Practice: Your Career Guide. Edited by Anne Hastie and Anne Stephenson. © 2008 Blackwell Publishing, ISBN: 978-1-4501-7070-3.

The GMC guidance has never been cited as the prime reason to teach by any teacher we have ever met, although supporting medical students and 'doctors in training' to become good practitioners is widely seen as an important professional responsibility.

Inspiration and continuing professional development

As the motivation for each individual is going to be different, one of the authors (AP) asked some of the enthusiastic teachers she knows why they had decided to go into teaching in general practice. The following quotes illustrate, better than any speculation, the myriad of reasons to teach.

> They teach me so much ... they bring excitement ... they value being valued ... it is the first time they have been valued as individuals in their career ... they flourish in the general practice.

> It is so wonderful when the eureka moment happens, when they see things in the new context of the patient and their life, not the disease. It is this reframing of their experience in a way that cannot be done by protocols that is so inspiring.

> The constant flow of fresh, unjaded faces into the practice stops us becoming complacent or cynical- the less experienced doctor continually asking "Why?" is the best stimulus to staying up to date and interested I know.

Teaching helps learning

> I teach in order to learn. I am now so old and stuck-in-my ways that I learn an enormous amount from those whom I am meant to be teaching. It started out as 'for the fun' – there is a great buzz in watching someone attain a skill or gain an understanding, and even more when you see it being put into practice – I fear if I gave up now I would rapidly fossilise!

The power of the apprenticeship model

The common theme described above inextricably links teaching with learning and this has been recently described in a chapter called 'How do we learn?' The question asked was: 'what's the best way to teach something difficult?'

> I think everyone has to find their own way to believe they can do something before they are likely to succeed. This could be watching, feeling, analysing or whatever – but if you've no self belief it's not likely to happen, no matter how much you study.

... yup, apart from copying someone I think you have to really want to succeed i.e. strong self-discipline as well. I usually crash from lack of this.

Watching videos, watching local hotshots. Just do it.

It's good to learn with a good teacher and the best teacher will vary from person to person. For me it's someone who will push me, but in such a way that I don't realize it is happening.

These quotes come from the UK windsurfing magazine *Boards*.[2] The descriptions are of a particular type of learning and teaching that has been called the apprenticeship model and could have been made by any GP registrar except perhaps 'crash' and 'local hotshot'! Teaching in primary care is uniquely placed to provide this form of apprenticeship learning. In undergraduate training there is normally one apprenticeship-type attachment of 4–8 weeks near the end of the undergraduate curriculum and in postgraduate training GP teachers (trainers) are usually allocated one GP registrar to their practice for a year.

Supporting professional transition

The close relationship that can ensue may be vital to support the change from medical school to being a new doctor; or from working in hospital posts and the acute care of hospital medicine to the long-term, ongoing brief interventions that make up so much of general practice. This is beautifully described by Iona Heath as 'the mystery of general practice'.[3] How do you teach or help the change from a medical student, who is used to being told what to do, to the more independent foundation doctor who has to start taking responsibility for patient care? How do you help young doctors in hospital medicine, used to doing all the 'right' tests and having someone else making a lot of the management decisions, suddenly cope with being alone with patients who do not come in with well-defined illness but have to be assessed in 10–15 minutes? Some doctors love taking on more responsibility immediately, but others need a lot of support. No one describes the role of the general practice teacher better than Roger Neighbour in *The Inner Apprentice*.[4] The analogy of the safety boat and life jacket needed in teaching windsurfing to allow learning implies the facility to make mistakes in a supportive and safe environment, i.e. the training practice. Some trainers describe the trainer–registrar relationship as unique, one to one, with modelling as a major influence on the development of the learner.

Studies of undergraduate GP teachers[5–7] mirror findings from postgraduate teachers, reporting contact with enthusiastic and questioning students, improved clinical practice and teaching skills, an increase in peer and professional support, increased time with patients and an improved image of general practice as positive outcomes. Teachers also value facilitating students' personal and professional development, a good experience encouraging students to enter general practice, of particular importance in the more deprived and urban environments. A lack of time and space, lack of financial reward, lack of flexibility, lack of confidence to teach and adverse effects on the teachers' time for patient care are perceived drawbacks of teaching undergraduate medical curricula. In spite of this in 2001 over one-third of general practices (about 3900) in the United Kingdom were involved in community-based undergraduate medical teaching[8] and at that time departments of general practice and primary care contributed an average of 9% of all undergraduate teaching in UK medical schools. With increases in student numbers the demands on undergraduate teachers and the number involved in teaching medical students are rising and, for a good practice, the opportunities for teaching medical students are many.

What do we teach in primary care?

General practice based medical education provides a multitude of teaching opportunities for educators and learning opportunities for students and doctors in training. The learning environment of primary care is a rich resource where students can learn about patient and population-centred care, whole person medicine, environmental, political, social and psychological factors affecting health, history taking and examination skills, the use of investigations, diagnosis, prescribing, the management of common conditions (acute and long-term, serious and non-serious), treating people at home, health promotion, continuity of care, team care, the range of services available and how to access them, healthcare law and ethics: the list is endless.[9] In postgraduate training the new curriculum for general practice training contains over 400 pages. In these times of large student numbers general practice placements provide individual attention and small group work, the general practice environment lending itself to professional development, and learning about communicating with patients and colleagues and having individual tuition in learning the skills required to be a doctor. Often it is in general practice that struggling learners are picked up and remedial work instituted. Apprenticeship models give the learner opportunities to consolidate and integrate their learning, develop their weaker areas and help teachers discern whether or not they are ready to go to the next stage of responsibility. Undergraduate and postgraduate teaching allows the teacher to support the medical student or young doctor in the transition between acute hospital medicine and looking after the extraordinary assortment of people and problems that make up the working day in general practice, including the realisation that many patients do not have a clear-cut diagnosis. Teaching the skill of rapid clinical assessment alongside the management of chronic disease is not straightforward and requires a particular skill in assessing what the learner already knows and what she doesn't. Teaching doctors-in-training how to manage uncertainty on their own is never easy and requires specific training.

How to become a teacher?

The career choices for teaching in general practice have never been straightforward but the following options illustrate the possibilities.

Undergraduate teaching
- Community-based undergraduate teachers attend the programme of teacher training events provided by the department for which they teach. (Some courses are run in collaboration with the local deanery.) They are also encouraged to seek certificates, diplomas and degrees in medical education.
- University-based academic teaching posts range from programme assistants, course leads, teaching fellows and senior teaching fellows, lecturers and senior lecturers, to directors and professors. Academics involved in developing and leading undergraduate teaching programmes are encouraged to seek postgraduate qualifications in education. Some are also required to do educational research and publish in peer-reviewed journals and this is increasingly a requirement of teaching posts.

Postgraduate general practice training
- Clinical supervisors need to attend an introductory training course.
- Trainers need to complete a postgraduate certificate in primary care education.
- Programme directors, senior lecturers/lecturers/formerly course organisers, are now encouraged to have postgraduate qualifications.
- Associate directors – as for programme directors.

At first sight these lists might seem a developmental hierarchy, but some community-based undergraduate teachers or clinical supervisors may have more teaching skills than an associate director, who acts as an educational manager, or university-based academic. The more experienced the teacher the more relevant are the higher order skills of providing support while at the same time being challenging. Some go on to take master's level courses in medical education or medical leadership. However a large number of those in the higher echelons of university departments and deaneries found themselves there through a love and belief in the importance of teaching and learning.

Historically, for both undergraduate and postgraduate teaching, anyone in the United Kingdom who put themselves forward could attend a course for a few days and then start teaching if approved. It has become increasingly clear that the higher the standard of teaching the better outcome for the learner. With the new focus on accountability across all sectors of society it is more important than ever to be able to show that you are committed enough to have your knowledge and skills as a teacher academically validated. General practice is fortunate in that there has always been an acknowledgement that teaching future doctors is of paramount importance and is highly valued. (Sadly, the same commitment is not given to all staff in primary care and the battle to support practice nurse development is not yet won.) General practice has been relatively privileged compared to hospital medicine in the resources it has been able to put into teaching the teachers.

For undergraduate teachers each medical school has its own arrangements for teaching their teachers. Teacher training can come from departmental courses, some set up jointly with local deaneries or education training courses, diplomas and degrees developed by universities and medical schools. Departments of general practice hold briefing and training sessions specific to their community-based teaching programmes. As yet a teacher training certificate is not required for undergraduate teachers although teacher training courses will soon need to be nationally accredited and it will only be a matter of time before new teachers will need accreditation in order to teach (see the Higher Education Academy website, http://www.heacademy.ac.uk/, for more information). Undergraduate GP teachers are paid for their time and even though the levels of re-provision do not pay for the cover required to allow teaching to take place, the payments are much more reasonable than they were 10–15 years ago.

In postgraduate teaching, trainers are also paid for their supervision and even though this financial inducement is small it does recognise the responsibilities and duties of teaching new doctors. Trainers of GP registrars are now not approved for training without both obtaining a postgraduate certificate in education and reaching a set of standards in their own clinical behaviour and that of their practice team.[10] This is in comparison to hospital posts where the emphasis from the royal colleges is to support the physician as educator, but as at 2007, this approach is not compulsory and the uptake is variable.

Development from Modernising Medical Careers

Many general practice deaneries and medical schools responded with alacrity to the exciting opportunity offered by Modernising Medical Careers (MMC) to have 55% of all doctors in their second foundation year working for

4 months in general practice. It is something that many in general practice have wanted for years. The possibility of enhancing recruitment into general practice has always been one consequence, but the other possibility is equally attractive in allowing hospital career clinicians to see what general practice is all about with the hope of improving communication and understanding between primary and secondary care. Even with increasing medical student community placements in undergraduate curricula and 'taster' days in general practice you cannot fully experience the job until you have experienced fully booked surgeries, home visits where patients are assessed in less than optimal circumstances, and the varied day as described in Chapter 2.

Preparing to teach

The importance of the general practitioners who provide undergraduate and postgraduate teaching placements being suitable role models cannot be over-emphasised. How sad if some of the prejudices expressed in hospital about GPs playing golf every afternoon, or just seeing patients with sore throats, or knowing no medicine, or just caring about money are actually experienced in these short posts. Undergraduate departments provide teacher training and the London Deanery has provided a minimum of 2-day training for generic teaching skills and a 1-day course to look at the curriculum and the new assessment tools of the foundation programme to help develop new teachers for this role. The London Deanery has also been involved since 2004 with a novel collaboration with all five London undergraduate departments of general practice to provide this generic teachers' course in the belief that the core skills needed to teach all levels of learner from undergraduate medical student, student nurse, health visitor and postgraduates are the same. This has led to the first 'Introduction to Teaching in Primary Care' (ITTPC) course in 2005–2006. This involved a group of teachers from all these institutions to agree on a programme to start new teachers off on a journey that hopefully at the very least enthuses, but may end with a Masters in Medical Education and a lifelong passion for education. The tutor notes that follow are intended to give an illustration of this course. Every course is different, modified as a result of the experience of and reflection on the previous courses. The example shown here was developed just before the second year started and was an amalgam of the previous six courses held in 2005 and 2006. The difficulty in finding a common syllabus with the five undergraduate departments of general practice teachers and the postgraduate deanery teachers was surprisingly painless, but a large number of areas had to be excluded for a 2-day course to deliver what was generally felt essential by all involved in the collaboration (see Box 14.1).

Box 14.1 An Introduction to Teaching in Primary Care (ITTPC) – a course for new teachers

Overall aims: Introduction to generic skills of teaching and learning.

Intended learning from Day 1: Opportunity to undertake a 'learning needs analysis' as part of preparing for learner-centred teaching.

Intended learning from Day 2: Opportunity to practice giving feedback as part of learner-centred teaching; plus find out about the next steps as an educator.

Day 1

Welcome and introductions

Fears, fantasies and hopes

Introduction to the skills of an effective teacher and teaching methods

The educational paradigm: aims, methods, assessment

Didactic, socratic, heuristic and counselling teaching styles

Learning needs assessment 1

    Presentation and assessment of learning needs, individually and in pairs

Planning for teaching

Lunch

Teaching practice 1 (in small groups)

    Each person delivers a 5-minute teaching session on anything that they wish inside or outside medicine

Teaching practice 2 (in small groups)

    Finish teaching sessions and group review of lessons learnt

Learning needs assessment 2

    Learning needs as a teacher. Self-reflection, including lessons learned from Day 1

Day 2

Welcome and overview of the day

Review of pre-course reading

Giving feedback

Introduction to teaching consultation skills

Teaching practice 3 (in small groups)

    Teaching consultation skills with participants role-playing patients, doctors and teachers

Lunch

Teaching practice 4 (in small groups)

    Teaching medical students, the students providing the topics

Next steps in teaching

Reflection on what has been learned and completion of evaluation form

Close

> **Box 14.2** Medical learners in general practice
>
> Undergraduate medical students
> Foundation programme Year 2 Doctors (FP2)
> GP Registrars Specialty Training 1 and 2 (SP1 and 2)
> Refugee and EU Doctors
> Retainer Doctors
> Flexible Career Scheme Doctors GP retainers clinical attachments for doctors
>   whose performance gives career for concern

All those undertaking the ITTPC, if supported, can teach medical students or supervise out of hours GP registrars and supervise F2 doctors in their GP attachment. There are many other roles for these new teachers including supporting GP retainers and 'returners' and refugee doctors on induction programmes.

Opportunities to teach

There are many types of learner in primary care and Box 14.2 illustrates some of them. This list does not include support and training of practice managers, receptionists, practice nurses, minor illness nurses, nurse practitioners and nurses applying for the prescribing list.

Next steps for GP trainers and programme directors

Those enthused and ready for more after the introduction to teaching course need to think about their next steps. The importance of good teachers in these times of great change can only be emphasised by the increasing number of deaneries requiring all new trainers of GP registrars to have as a minimum requirement a Postgraduate Certificate of Education and membership of the Royal College of General Practitioners. It is interesting now to note the howls of outrage when compulsory postgraduate certification was introduced. Many course organisers and associate directors said that there would not be enough people coming forward to become GP trainers. The opposite has occurred in most areas with spare GP trainers now competing with clinical supervisors for F2 doctor supervision. A few critics said that academic accreditation was not appropriate for the pragmatic teaching that GP trainers provide. However, the vast majority of those who undertake a postgraduate certificate in education recognize the added value that academic perspectives can give to practical skills – 'there is nothing so practical as a good theory'.[11]

Most deaneries now run their own courses and an example of the London Deanery teaching course is outlined below, running since 1997 as an accredited postgraduate certificate in primary care education. It has expanded in the last 5 years to have two cohorts with entries in September and April of each year. The course is interprofessional and has a format that encourages group learning as the prime focus with no fixed time table but a flexible syllabus that tries to relate to the needs and wishes of the group. The aims and content of the programme are described in Box 14.3.

Box 14.3 Teaching the teachers (TTT), London Deanery[10]

Programme aims

This course aims to meet the broad educational needs of all teachers in primary care by evaluating critically:

 The principles of adult education

 Work-based self-directed learning

 Self- and peer-assessment for continuing professional development

Learning outcomes

To be able to:

 Design a curriculum appropriate to the needs of learners

 Analyse a range of educational methods and relate them to the principles of adult learning

 Critically evaluate your ability to provide learning support

 Identify and critically evaluate a range of assessment techniques and select and use them appropriately

 Reflect on your learning and develop a critical enquiry approach to your teaching practice

 Communicate effectively with those you are teaching and your peers

 Critically evaluate educational materials, such as publications, personal development plans and teaching sessions

Course content

Core topics identified from previous cohorts of students include:

 Introduction to learning in groups

 Models of the consultation

 Curriculum planning and syllabus setting

 Teaching methods

 Reflective practice

 Formative assessment and mentorship

 Learning needs analysis

Personal learning plans
Interprofessional working
Participants on previous courses have identified additional topics, which have
    varied from year to year, such as:
        Critical reading and evidence-based practice
        Time management
        Selection skills
        Advanced group learning
        Management skills/IT skills

The course can be a culture shock for many strategic learners who have been used to being 'told' what to do and when to do it all through their medical life. The following comments from students taken from the 2006–2007 prospectus illustrate the change that can take place during the course which covers an academic year with 12 taught days and reading and working in between those days. There is always a tension between being told what to learn and being supported to discover for yourself and develop into the 'lifelong learner'. This tension is as great for doctors becoming teachers as for medical students becoming doctors.

Stimulating, interactive, confidence-building

More encouraging and thought-provoking than any course I have
ever been on

Well-structured, good variety, lots of opportunity for reflection, good
'role models' for teachers

Helped me gain confidence when working and learning
interprofessionally. I would recommend this course to other trainers

Summary

This chapter has been devoted to those thousands of general practitioners working as trainers, clinical supervisors and undergraduate teachers doing their best to enthuse, cajole and infect their many learners in an extraordinary job with its own unique highs and lows. Frank McCourt in *Teacher Man*[12] sums up the teaching philosophy of many of them.

This is where the teacher turns serious and asks the Big Question:
What is education anyway? What are we doing in this school? You can

say you're trying to graduate so that you can go to college and prepare for a career. But, fellow students, it's more than that. I've had to ask myself what the hell I am doing in the classroom. I've worked out an equation for myself. On the left side of the blackboard I print a capital F; on the right side another capital F; I draw an arrow from left to right, from FEAR to FREEDOM. I don't think anyone achieves complete freedom, but what I am trying to do with you is drive fear into a corner.

References

1 General Medical Council (2001) *Good Medical Practice.* London: General Medical Council.
2 Article on 'How do we learn?' from *Boards magazine* on www.boards.co.uk
3 Heath I (1995) *The Mystery of General Practice.* London: Nuffield Provincial Hospitals Trust.
4 Neighbour R (1992) *The Inner Apprentice.* UK: Plymouth Petroc Press.
5 Gray J, Fine B (1997) General practitioner teaching in the community: a study of their teaching experience and interest in undergraduate teaching in the future. *British Journal of General Practice* **47**: 623–626.
6 Hartley S, Macfarlane F, Gantley M, Murray E (1999) Influence on general practitioners of teaching undergraduates: qualitative study of London general practitioner teachers. *British Medical Journal* **319**:168–171.
7 Mathers J, Parry J, Lewis, S, Greenfield S (2004) What impact will an increased number of teaching general practices have on patients, doctors and medical students? *Medical Education* **38**:1219–1228.
8 Society for Academic Primary Care. *New Century, New Challenges: A report from the Heads of Departments of General Practice and Primary Care in the Medical Schools of the United Kingdom.* http://www.sapc.ac.uk/docs/Mackenzie2.pdf (accessed 30 April 2007).
9 Stephenson A (ed.) (1998) *A Textbook of General Practice.* London: Arnold (2nd edition 2005).
10 London Deanery. *GP Training Guide.* http://www.londondeanery.ac.uk/general-practice/specialty-training-for-gp/gp-training-guide (accessed 17 May 2007).
11 Lewin K (1935) *A Dynamic Theory of Personality.* New York: McGraw-Hill.
12 McCourt F (2005) *Teacher Man.* London: Fourth Estate.

Chapter 15 **Professional values**

John Spicer

What are values, and what values should a general practitioner possess?

Introduction

When we speak of 'values' in connection with the professional role of general practitioners (GPs) it is easy to get confused about the meaning of the word, as it is often mixed up with words such as 'standards' or 'rules'. So in this chapter I am going to start by clearing up the meanings of all these terms, and then discuss why GPs should actually possess any values at all. In doing so I will identify differences between general practice (or primary care) and hospital care, where such values may be a little different.

As described in the rest of this book, the modern GP is a particular kind of doctor compared to how he was 50 years ago. He is much less likely to be male, and thus more likely to be a 'she'. She will work in a team of various kinds of health care professionals, who collectively and individually offer a much wider range of care to patients than was the case in the past. She will have undergone a formal training programme for general practice and that will include the learning of all the skills necessary to do the job. She may well be teaching students or other learners in the practice. Those aspects are detailed elsewhere in this book. What has not changed, for GPs, is the continuing relationship with patients over time, over many episodes of illness, and in the context of their patients within their families: that is the core of general practice. These factors, above all, affect the values that GPs should possess.

Choosing General Practice: Your Career Guide. Edited by Anne Hastie and Anne Stephenson. © 2008 Blackwell Publishing, ISBN: 978-1-4501-7070-3.

Values, standards and rules

So what does a *value* mean? Differing definitions abound, but the most commonly stated is that something is valuable if it is desirable, useful or of quality. In contrast, a *standard* is what might be expected or required. It is a more formal quality, and for GPs could be described as an acceptable level of knowledge or skill for the job. *Rules* are the compulsory frameworks that GPs must take account of in their day-to-day practice.

Let's try and explain those differences a little more: when a GP sees her patients every day, she will work under several systems of rules. There is a legal background, and clearly she cannot disobey any law concerning the delivery of care. An example of this is the rather complex law surrounding consent: if she prescribes a medicine then she must ensure that the patient understands the nature and purpose of the medicine she is suggesting, that the patient can actually understand its need and is making a free choice to accept the treatment. In the United Kingdom this law of consent is mainly what is known as *common* law (or case law), as it comes to us from the interpretation of cases in the courts, rather than from Acts of Parliament as *statute* law is.

There are also professional rules under which GPs must operate, and these are defined in the United Kingdom by the General Medical Council (GMC). At the time of writing the GMC define these rules to interpret and apply the law, offering guidance to all doctors in their day-to-day clinical work. In the case of consent there is succinct and clear guidance on offer.

It is expected that GPs should follow the rules as described above: anything less would be considered to be below the standard of acceptable practice in the United Kingdom.

Finally, moral rules concern those aspects of practice that are separate from the law or any professional rules. Morality is all about differentiating what is right from what is wrong. Some GPs, for example, feel that offering contraception to young patients is morally appropriate and some don't. It is a personal decision, based on one's own sense of what is right. That sense may be informed by intuition, reflection, discussion or even by the membership of a particular religion.

Sources of medical rules

- The law
- Professional rules
- Moral rules

Having clarified these meanings, we can begin to describe in more detail what a value is and how they relate to GPs in general. I have already stated that something is valuable if is of quality or useful, but as with all definitions there is a problem of scope. Something that one GP might find to be useful in dealing with her patients may not be so useful to another, and it might be asked as to whether it is really the usefulness to the patient that matters. There are at least two ways of getting at this problem: firstly, by considering the moral, or ethical, frameworks that are relevant, and secondly by differentiating evidence-based practice from value-based practice.

Ethics and the GP

It has been said that the 'stuff' of general practice is the consultation between GP and patient. It is not a derogatory phrase, though it might appear so, but really articulates the primacy of the interaction between the two parties. They come together for all sorts of reasons, but primarily for the GP to offer some alleviation of suffering, which may be physical, social, psychological or a combination of all. She will do that usually in the context of a long-term relationship with that patient, knowing the family or social milieu and addressing all the aspects of the patient's health (the holistic view). It is clearly a complex task to undertake.

Every such consultation will contain issues of right and wrong: moral issues. For the record, I will consider the words moral and ethical almost interchangeable. It isn't strictly true but will suffice for now. To lend some weight to the statement about the universality of general practice ethics, look at these questions or dilemmas that have arisen from the every day work of one GP:

Box 15.1 Some every day ethical dilemmas

1 A patient wants to switch his insulin over to a non-porcine insulin for religious reasons.

2 A patient wants a prescription for a medicine that has no scientific evidence for its usefulness.

3 A patient asks to discuss his mother's failing mental health without her knowledge of the discussion.

4 A patient declines a medicine that the GP knows will ease his pain because he believes it harmful.

5 A patient wants to be referred to a hospital for which there is no agreed referral contract within the NHS.

6 A patient tries to persuade the GP to remove a skin lesion on her face despite the risk of scarring.

7 A patient insists on a GP prescribing a new drug that has not yet entered the Primary Care Trust (PCT) formulary.

8 A patient of intellectual impairment declines an injection intended to prevent tetanus after a minor injury.

9 A parent asks for a clinically irrelevant X-ray of her child.

None of these cases are at the scientific cutting edge but they all contain ethical material, and they are certainly every day work for GPs. They purposefully illustrate situations where there is, or might be, dissent between doctor and patient. Take the first example: the patient is unwilling to consider porcine insulin as his religion, he believes, forbids its use. In some religions, pigs are held to be unclean animals and those revealed texts describe these objections in more detail. We must assume that this religious dimension informs the patient's personal morality. For him, it is a moral value that he refrains from eating pork, or injecting porcine insulin. It really doesn't matter if the GP sees things differently: that is the patient's perspective and should be respected.

In sorting out the clinical dilemma both GP and patient should be aware of their, perhaps, contrary views. As it happens most insulin now is of human type so the patient with a religious objection can be easily accommodated. That was not the case when most insulin was mainly of pork type.

If the religious argument is ignored, then another moral perspective is given by the consequences of the decision. While human insulin was not available, patients with such a religious objection found themselves in a difficult situation. Was it morally right to refuse pork insulin even though health would inevitably suffer, perhaps to the point of death?

Clearly in this case, the outcome of a religious decision to refuse a potentially life-saving medication would be adverse, and therefore of itself arguably morally wrong. In fact, religious authorities often soften moral rules of this type in the presence of medical reasons and allow a 'utilitarian', as it is known, decision to permit such a treatment. As such, the value of positive outcome is the overriding value. Nonetheless, the value to the patient of holding to his religious belief that excludes use of porcine products is useful, desirable and of quality. It is also a reflection of religious duty as defined by those in the religion who define it thus, something that could be similarly described.

In the last example, no doubt the GP will have a discussion with the parent who is requesting what she feels to be an X-ray without utility. The GP's opinion is probably that investigations of this type are potentially a waste of scarce resources and will not benefit or might harm the patient. Clearly the parent believes that some benefit will accrue to the child, perhaps until the discussion is had. He might have some particular respect for what he believes to be the value of the X-ray in revealing disease. On the other hand the GP may have access to clinically based evidence to support her position.

Put like this, it sounds as if the two points of view cannot be drawn together and a compromise reached, but actually the GP is in a good position to bring that about. It is part of her skills as a GP to negotiate with the parent, to find out exactly why he thinks as he does and to discover the values that he brings to the conversation. It is likely that the parent attaches some considerable value to the technology of the X-ray machine, not understanding its limitations. So there is an element to the conversation about *evidence,* or the scientific basis of the X-ray: what it can and cannot show. There is also an element about *value,* or what the GP and parent hold to be important in the discussion.

There is something else too: the discussion between GP and parent is a moral discussion, as it will include elements that both people consider to be about right and wrong. Perhaps the doctor is very conscious of costs, of the financial value of the investigation they are talking about. Perhaps the parent considers it his right to have an X-ray when he wants one. This element is all about the *ethical process* of the discussion. It might not be obvious, or even known to the GP and parent, but it is there. The discussion, reasoning and conclusions are of ethical value in themselves.

Key values for the GP

We have seen that values for GPs and patients may happily coincide, but may not. The next thing to consider is whether we can define a set of values that GPs should have: what is termed *normative* or *stipulative*. There are many possible values that could be generated under this heading and the following is a guide to do it, rather than a somewhat cold list. There are powerful arguments that GPs should attach value to the following, in no particular order:

Box 15.2 Core GP values

- Maintaining their knowledge and skills through continuing education
- Working in the 'best interests' of their patients
- Respecting their patients decisions
- Being aware of their own values and attitudes
- Reasoning through clinical ethical dilemmas
- Being respectful of differences between patients
- Working in medical and multidisciplinary teams
- Caring for patients in their own environments
- Caring for patients over time
- Caring for patients within their families
- Considering the whole population of their patients, as well as individuals.

This list is not exhaustive and various GPs might attach more importance to one than another. However, any GP in the United Kingdom (and also elsewhere) will find it impossible to practice successfully, or even lawfully, without some incorporation of these attributes into day-to-day work. There are two particular strands of moral knowledge that inform such a list.

Firstly, there is *virtue ethics*, which sounds rather idealised in that form. In essence, virtue ethics suggests that one way of deciding what is right and wrong is to focus on the person doing the deciding, rather than the thing that is to be decided. So in the clinical examples in Box 15.1, we might consider the attributes of the GP that make it easier for her to reach the 'right' decision in each case. In some examples, she would usefully bring to bear sensitivity, in others courage and in others a willingness to compromise.

So what she would be demonstrating is a particular set of personal attributes that help bring about an ethically sound outcome to the decision. This way of looking at ethics has a long history: in fact, the GP who looked at ethics in this way would be standing on the shoulders of Hippocrates, who in writing his famous oath described good medical practice in terms of the virtues of its practitioners. Clearly what we could describe as virtuous attributes (rather than vicious) are closely related to the list of appropriate values above.

Secondly, there is the notion of *professionalism* and what might be considered to be professional values in themselves. The term professional is often used rather imprecisely and applied among others, to lawyers, plumbers, soldiers and members of the oldest profession. Nonetheless, doctors in general and GPs in particular would no doubt describe themselves as professionals too. What might this description mean? Over the years, many theorists have tackled this issue and the following characteristics are suggested as a distillation of that work: professionals are generally held to be members of a professional *organisation* which promotes the value of their work. They have an *esoteric*, or specialised, knowledge and language that describes their work. There is some notion of *duty* to their clients which may go beyond what is loosely described as contracted for. They recognise a value in continuing learning to *maintain* their work skills. They are in some way *licensed* by the state or other body. To some extent they work *autonomously*.

These criteria are all represented in the day-to-day work of the twenty-first century European GP. They will vary between countries, and even within countries, but those key professional issues endure.

Readers will have spotted that the idealised list of key GP values in Box 15.2 is therefore a synthesis of three themes: *virtues*, or personal attributes; *professional* attributes and the particular qualities relevant to primary care. For example, the care of any of the patients in Box 15.1 should necessarily require the GP to continue to learn, the motivation to do it, and its application to the case in question. In addition, the GP should respect the patient's values,

> **Box 15.3** A complex case
>
> Mrs Bloggs is 91 and fiercely independent. She lives at home on her own, despite hypothyroidism, hypertension, widespread osteoarthrosis, glaucoma and type 2 diabetes. She is immobile, and requires carers to help her with all the activities of daily living. She listens to the radio or TV most of the day, and reads the newspapers with a large magnifying glass. Her only family is a son who lives in another town and with whom she has no contact. One day she falls out of her chair, and the GP attends at the request of the care staff. They feel Mrs Bloggs should be admitted to hospital, though she disagrees loudly. A muscular injury is suspected. The GP wonders what she should do?

relating them to her own knowledge of the patient over many consultations, as a professional skill.

Doctors in secondary care have no less a set of professional skills and attributes, but it is generally concentrated in smaller, more detailed areas of knowledge and over shorter time scales: usually within a hospital admission and follow-up. Specialist medical care would therefore appeal to those who are interested in dealing in a smaller segment of medicine to greater depth than that of a GP.

Slightly confusingly in learning the skills and values of UK general practice, trainees are called specialist trainees in general practice. The value of clarity and precision in use of language seems, in this context, to be elusive.

Summary

This chapter has dealt with some of the values important to patients, and also the values relevant to the professional practice of primary care. It is a necessarily brief introduction to a complex subject, but if its complexities appeal to you, then general practice could well be for you. As an exercise, see if in this real scenario, in box 15.3 you can speculate as to the patient's and the GP's values.

Further reading

If readers are considering a career in general practice and wish to know more about this field then there are some excellent sources in the public domain.
- *The Royal College of General Practitioners Curriculum* has a long section on Values Based Practice (s3.3) and is at http://www.rcgp.org.uk/

PDF/curr_3_3_Ethics_2006.pdf. All these themes are dealt with in more detail and the material is a key part of the learning agenda for GPs in training.

* *Towards a Philosophy of General Practice:A Study of the Virtuous Practitioner* by Peter Toon (Occasional Paper No. 78 RCGP) is a full exploration of the place of virtue theory in modern day general practice.

* In *Practical Ethics for General Practice,* Wendy Rogers and Annette Braunack-Mayer have wonderfully described the larger area of GP ethics as a whole. It is recommended for further reading (Oxford University Press 2004 ISBN 978019852042).

* The UK General Medical Council produces a series of leaflets containing advice about the duties of doctors and specific advice on consent, management, confidentiality and many others. Essentially these are professional rules statements.

* The *Journal of Medical Ethics,* published in the United Kingdom, paints a larger picture still: across primary and secondary care, and linked to ethical issues beyond health care. Much material is easily readable for the general clinical reader, though some is not.

* EURACT, the Academy of European Teacher in General Practice and Family Medicine, has produced a set of definitions and statements about the activity of the modern GP. It is the foundation of the new RCGP curriculum and full of useful material in this area (see http://www.euract.org/html/page03f.shtml).

Chapter 16 **General practitioners with special interests**

Roger Jones

Background

Before the foundation of the College of General Practitioners in 1952 and the introduction of mandatory vocational training in the 1960s, entrance to general practice was relatively uncontrolled. It was possible for recent medical graduates to go into practice without specific training, and for doctors who had spent time in hospital medicine to move straight into a post in general practice, bringing with them skills and expertise learnt in medicine, surgery, obstetrics and gynaecology, anaesthesia and other specialities. At this time, and well into the 1980s, general practitioner hospitals, numbering around 300 in England, Wales and Scotland, were in their heyday, and the general practitioner surgeon and obstetrician were well-recognised figures on the primary care landscape. Low-risk obstetrics and a range of surgical procedures conducted under general anaesthetic were commonly undertaken by general practitioners in the community, and some pioneers introduced community-based gastrointestinal endoscopy and other procedures more typically undertaken in hospital settings. General practitioners in possession of FRCS and MRCOG qualifications were not unusual, and many well-trained general practitioner anaesthetists supported their activities.

As well as contributing to the work of general practitioner and community hospitals, many GPs practising in rural and remote areas were required to possess expertise and skills which enabled them to deal with acute medical, surgical and obstetric emergencies because of the long distances between their surgeries and the nearest district hospital. In addition, many general practitioners with hospital experience continued their links with their hospital through appointments as clinical assistants, working in hospital outpatient departments and often running specialist clinics, with consultant supervision

---

Choosing General Practice: Your Career Guide. Edited by Anne Hastie and Anne Stephenson. © 2008 Blackwell Publishing, ISBN: 978-1-4501-7070-3.

in district general as well as community hospitals in a range of medical and surgical sub-specialities. Arrangements for accreditation and clinical governance were poorly developed at this time, although there is some evidence that these 'GP specialists' were providing a cost-effective and clinically sound contribution to medical care which was more convenient for patients and relieved some of the pressures on referral to district general hospitals.[1,2] Engagement in this kind of work had the undoubted advantage of providing a more varied job description for general practitioners and also contributed to improved communication between them and the specialists in their local district hospital.

With the advent of vocational training, limited to 2 years of hospital experience and a year in an 'apprenticeship' role in general practice, the number of doctors with substantial hospital experience entering general practice began to dwindle, and at the same time the role and cost-effectiveness of general practitioner and community hospitals was coming under increasing scrutiny by health authorities. The days of the swashbuckling general practitioner surgeon were numbered.

Recent developments

Health policy developments over the last few years have, however, seen a renaissance of interest in both community hospitals and in the role of general practitioners with special clinical interests. The recently-published Government White Paper on the extension of medical care into the community 'Our Health, Our Care, Our Say'[3] has charged Primary Care Trusts (PCTs) to review the role of general practitioner hospitals in their health economies, and the NHS Plan,[4] published in 2000, had identified the importance of developing a cadre of general practitioners with special clinical interests potentially able to make an impact on access to hospital care in long waiting-list specialities such as ENT, orthopaedics, ophthalmology and dermatology. The general practitioner with a special clinical interest was back, although in a more highly regulated form than before.

Special interests

It appears, however, that vocational training had not inhibited general practitioners from pursuing special interests outside their standard General Medical Services contracts. In 2001 a national, cross-sectional survey of 931 general practitioners, selected at random from one health authority within each of the eight English health regions, revealed that over 70% of the respondents had at least one clinical interest, covering over 60 different clinical topics.[5]

Table 16.1 Top 10 clinical interests and clinical sessions of respondents ($n = 390$)

Clinical interests ($n = 282$)			Clinical sessions ($n = 152$)		
	n	%		n	%
Diabetes	57	20	Diabetes	26	17
Dermatology	41	15	Dermatology	16	11
Family planning	34	12	Minor surgery	13	9
Paediatrics	25	9	Family planning	12	8
Gynaecology	25	9	Occupational health	11	7
Minor surgery	23	8	Gynaecology	8	5
Cardiology	20	7	Cardiology	7	5
Psychiatry	18	6	Endoscopy	6	4
Acupuncture	18	6	Acupuncture	6	4
Drug addiction	17	6	Geriatrics, orthopaedics, Paediatrics, palliative care sports medicine	5	3

The most frequently mentioned of these were diabetes (20%), dermatology (15%), family planning (12%), paediatrics (9%), gynaecology (9%), minor surgery (8%), cardiology (7%), psychiatry (6%), acupuncture (6%) and drug addiction (6%). More than one-third of the GPs responding to this survey reported undertaking clinical sessions in these areas of particular clinical interest. This means that, even if none of the non-responders to the survey did any clinical sessions at all, around 16% (approximately 4000) of all GPs in England were involved in one or more clinical sessions in areas of special interests. Interestingly, this figure varied from 11% in London to 22% in the West Midlands, Wales and the South West. Over half of these sessions were undertaken outside health centre and practice premises. About a third were performed in acute hospitals, and about 10% each in community trusts, community hospitals and other settings. The contractual arrangements under which these GPs were working were variable, with about one-third working as clinical assistants and a fifth as hospital practitioners, with the remainder working under a variety of contractual arrangements. The clinical sessions in areas of special interest undertaken by these GPs are shown in the table, with diabetes, dermatology, minor surgery, family planning and occupational health being the most frequently reported special interests (Table 16.1).

In the survey GPs were asked to indicate why they were doing this extra work. They said that the maintenance of special interests provided variety and added interest to their professional life, whilst at the same time offering better and more accessible services for their patients. Of particular note was the finding of considerable mismatch between the clinical topics in which GPs

were conducting these sessions and the long waiting-list specialities identified in the NHS Plan for the development of GPs with special interests
(GPwSIs).

Specialist societies

Over the last 20 years, long before the NHS Plan identified the importance
of GPwSIs, general practitioners with particular clinical expertise and experience had begun to form themselves into a number of specialist societies.
The first of these was the Primary Care Society for Gastroenterology (PCSG),
founded in 1986, and aiming to provide a focus for clinical, research and educational aspects of gastroenterology.[6] The majority of the members of PCSG
were GP endoscopists – doctors who had trained in endoscopy in their hospital careers and had decided to continue to use their expertise by providing
endoscopy services in their localities, based either in their own practices or,
more frequently, in general practitioner hospitals or in hospital outpatient
departments. The PCSG now has a membership of around 450, the majority of whom are GP endoscopists. The Society has been active in developing
guidelines for the management of a range of gastrointestinal problems, including irritable bowel syndrome, coeliac disease, dyspepsia and the early
identification of colorectal cancer, and has contributed to the appreciation by
gastroenterology specialists of the important contribution made by general
practitioners working in primary care gastroenterology. The Society has also
been instrumental in re-defining the contractual arrangements under which
GPwSIs in gastroenterology are employed. In the past most had been employed under the Clinical Assistant grade arrangements, which provided low
levels of remuneration, poor job security and little opportunity for professional development. Many of these GPs were able to transfer to the Hospital
Practitioner grade, which offered better remuneration and job security, as
well as providing study leave and professional developmental opportunities.
Many are now employed as GPwSIs in gastroenterology. Some have taken a
much more entrepreneurial line with their PCT, and have been able to negotiate favourable contracts with PCTs for the provision of community-based
endoscopy services, often sited in purpose-converted practice premises.

Many other primary care specialist societies have developed over the last
10–15 years, representing GPwSIs in cardiology, rheumatology, dermatology,
asthma, mental health and other specialist areas. An umbrella organisation,
the UK Federation of Primary Care Specialist Societies, has been formed
and now holds an annual conference providing a focus for the work of these
groups. There is a list of contact details for these societies at the end of this
chapter.

Box 16.1 Areas considered most likely to be priorities in terms of national programmes or services with significant access problems

- Cardiology
- Care of the elderly
- Diabetes
- Palliative care and cancer
- Mental health (including substance misuse)
- Dermatology
- Musculoskeletal medicine
- Women and child health, including sexual health
- Ear, nose and throat
- Care for the homeless, asylum seekers, travellers and others who find access to traditional health services difficult
- Other procedures suitable for community setting (endoscopy, cystoscopy, echocardiography, vasectomy, etc.)

General practitioners with special interests

The formalisation of GPwSIs has come through the recommendations of the 2000 NHS Plan, which specified the need to develop at least 1000 GPwSIs working in the community and providing services as an alternative to hospital referral in selected areas. The Department of Health (DH) has worked closely with the Royal College of General Practitioners to provide guidance on the job descriptions, accreditation and clinical governance aspects of GPwSIs in a number of areas, listed in Box 16.1. PCTs have responded variably to this policy initiative. In some parts of the country GPwSI posts have been set up specifically to enhance recruitment and retention, by providing a varied portfolio of work for GPs. In other areas GPwSI services have been developed to plug gaps in the provision of specialist services and to improve access for patients, often in 'niche' areas such as substance abuse, refugee health and the health care of the homeless and those with serious mental illness. The DH guidance on the process of establishing a GPwSI service is shown in Figure 16.1.

Evaluation of GPwSI services

The research into and evaluation of GPwSI services is still fairly thin. Two reports of a randomised controlled trial of GPwSI services in dermatology in the west of England[7,8] have indicated that whilst clinical outcomes are equivalent and patient satisfaction at least as good with GPwSI services compared with hospital clinics, the costs of providing these services are

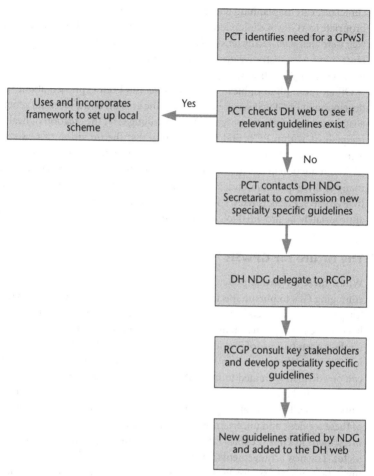

Figure 16.1 How a PCT sets up a GPSI scheme (*DH National Development Group)

substantially greater than those incurred in consultant clinics. In another research study, examining the working of a number of GPwSI clinics providing services in dermatology, cardiology, mental health and orthopaedics, some of other potential problems were identified, including poor use of information systems with consequent difficulties in auditing services, wide variations in standards of clinical governance, accreditation and continuing professional development, and also considerable variation in relationships between primary and secondary care.[9] Successful GPwSI services were characterised by strong support from both primary and secondary care managers and clinicians, careful planning and careful definition of the case-mix most appropriate to a GPwSI clinic. Conversely, GPwSI services which were faring less well were characterised by tensions between general practitioners and consultants, poor administrative arrangements and uncertainty about the criteria for referral of patients to GP specialists.

Other, more philosophical, concerns have also been expressed about the development of GPwSI services, including the erosion of the essential generalist function of GPs, the potential for de-skilling GPs, the creation of health inequalities within PCTs and the possibility that the provision of new services might simply lead to an escalation of patient referrals, rather than the desired reduction in referral to specialists. More research is needed to answer many of these questions and, in particular, to determine whether investment by PCTs in GPwSIs is truly cost-effective, or whether funding should more appropriately be provided to expand hospital facilities.[10]

The future for GPwSIs

Whilst there are strong policy and professional arguments in favour of encouraging GPs to pursue special interests and to provide additional services for patients, there is concern about whether a 'one size fits all' approach is likely to be appropriate. Many GPs currently working as GPwSIs have taken up their posts because of previous experience and expertise in particular clinical areas, and there must be questions about how new generations of GPwSIs can be adequately trained to move into these posts as doctors move on and retire. Clinical governance issues of certification and re-validation will continue to arise. There are also significant questions about the cost-effectiveness of these services, and uncertainty about whether it is appropriate to continue investment in GPwSI clinics rather than expanding capacity in the hospital sector. The new arrangements for Practice Based Commissioning provide an important mechanism for PCTs to identify gaps in services which can most appropriately be filled by GPs providing this level of intermediate care, and PCTs will need to look carefully at the best ways of harnessing the enthusiasms of GPs with particular clinical skills and to work creatively with colleagues in hospital medicine to ensure that investment in these services is appropriate and cost-effective.

Federation of British Primary Care Societies

General Practice Airways Group.
    www.gpiag.org
The Primary Care Cardiovascular Society.
    www.pccs.org.uk

Primary Care Dermatology Society.
www.pcds.org.uk
Primary Care Diabetes UK.
www.diabetes.org.uk
Primary Care Mental Health and Education.
www.primhe.org
The Primary Care Rheumatology Society.
www.pcrsociety.org.uk
Primary Care Society for Gastroenterology.
www.pcsg.org.uk

References

1 O'Caithan A, Brazier JE, Milner PC, Fall M (1992) Cost effectiveness of minor surgery in general practice: a prospective comparison with hospital practice. *British Journal of General Practice* **42**: 13–17.

2 Hakkaart-van Roijen L, Moll van Charante EP, Bindels PJ, et al. (2004) A cost study of a general practitioner hospital in the Netherlands. *European Journal of General Practice* **10**: 45–49.

3 Department of Health (2006) *Our Health, Our Care, Our Say: A New Direction for Community Services.* London: Stationery Office.

4 Secretary of State for Health (2000) *The NHS Plan: A Plan for Investment, a Plan for Reform.* London: Stationery Office.

5 Jones R, Bartholomew J (2002) General practitioners with special clinical interests: a cross-sectional survey. *British Journal of General Practice* **52**: 833–834.

6 http://www.pcsg.org.uk/

7 Salisbury C, Noble A, Horrocks S, et al. (2005) Evaluation of a general practitioner with special interest service for dermatology: randomised controlled trial. *British Medical Journal* **331**: 1441–1446.

8 Coast J, Noble S, Noble A, et al. (2005) Economic evaluation of a general practitioner with special interests led dermatology service in primary care. *British Medical Journal* **331**: 1444–1449.

9 Rosen R, Jones R, Tomlin Z, Cavanagh M-R (2005) Evaluation of general practitioners with special interests: access, cost evaluation and satisfaction with services. *NCCSDO* August 2005 (Revised January 2006).

10 Jones R, Rosen R, Tomlin Z, Cavanagh M-R, Oxley D (2006) General practitioners with special interests: evolution and evaluation. *Journal of Health Services Research & Policy* **11**: 106–109.

Chapter 17 **Leadership and management**

Julia Whiteman

Introduction

You are in your surgery and your next patient comes in but before you can start the consultation he begins by complaining that it took 3 days to get through on the phone to make this appointment, there is nowhere to park in the car park as usual because people who are not patients use it as free parking for the railway station, he is being seen 40 minutes after the appointment time and 'There's someone out in the waiting room who doesn't look at all well. He has gone all grey and sweaty!' He then launches into what he wants from you – a National Insurance Certificate for his bad back, the other doctors in the practice have refused to issue a further one, so he has come back to you as you gave him one before.

Hopefully all these issues coming together is not typical of many consultations taking place in GP surgeries as a GP receiving any one of the pieces of information in the previous paragraph would realise that he or she was in a challenging situation. But I hope it encapsulates something of the potential of what can happen in the normal working day of a GP, which calls upon a broader range of knowledge and skills than the purely clinical ones associated with being a doctor.

Turn the first paragraph around. The patient comes in and compliments you on how easy it is to make an appointment since the new telephone system has been introduced. He says that the new sign politely asking people not to use the car parking spaces unless they are seeing someone at the practice and the system for recording car registration numbers at reception has really worked. There is always room for disabled parking now. The information in the practice newsletter about the appointment system time slots and the difference between longer booked appointments and emergency appointments

Choosing General Practice: Your Career Guide. Edited by Anne Hastie and Anne Stephenson. © 2008 Blackwell Publishing, ISBN: 978-1-4501-7070-3.

has helped to make things run on time. 'And your receptionists were so quick to spot that that man was not well! He did look grey! Your nurse was so efficient and professional. He obviously needed to be seen urgently. We all appreciated being informed about the delay. Some people did rebook their appointments. Wasn't the ambulance quick? I do hope he will be OK!'

Then, in this ideal world, the patient tells you that he understands why you did not agree to keep signing him off from work about his bad back, he has been doing the exercises, feels much better and has even found a part-time job. He would like to take up your offer for a referral to physiotherapy.

This chapter will look at the management processes occurring behind the services offered by GPs and their primary care teams to patients, and the part that a GP might play in influencing those services.

Historical context

The notion of multi-professional participation in patient care[1] with clear lines of responsibility and influence for all members of the primary health care team only really became established in the 1990s.[2] The National Health Service (NHS) was originally set up in 1948 following the publication during the Second World War of the Beveridge Report.[3] It is not surprising therefore that the structure and function of the newly formed NHS was strongly linked to the needs of a country at war, namely for a healthy community of young men who could become soldiers and civilians who were able to live under the stress and demands of war with greater demands on their physical health and strength. Doctors were cast as the clear and unquestionable leaders who were to be obeyed by both staff and patients alike.

With the formation of the NHS important differences were established between doctors working in hospitals and those working in the community as GPs. Doctors working as GPs were given the status of independent contractors whilst hospital consultants were offered employment contracts with the NHS. Therein lays the basis of the working status of GPs who are established as clinicians but working in practices that are run as small businesses with the GPs in charge. A further difference between GPs and doctors working in the hospital setting was that doctors pursuing a career in hospital medicine were part of a structured training programme leading to a consultancy. Successful completion of a doctor's training programme in hospital medicine was dependent on passing Royal College examinations relevant to the speciality. On the other hand, it was not until the 1970s that vocational training was established for GPs and then not until the 1990s that an end-point assessment was introduced for GPs completing training. It is therefore not surprising that with the formation of the NHS GPs were not held in the same high regard as hospital doctors by both the profession and public alike.

During the 1980s and 1990s there was considerable change in the organisation of the health service and the way that patient care was delivered. The Griffiths Report[4] was instrumental in promoting clinicians as managers as well as leaders in the health service, but it was the NHS and Community Care Act in 1990 that brought together the different professions from medicine, nursing and social services together. The Act established new strategic working patterns within financial frameworks whereby primary care purchased services from secondary care, social services and community trusts, working within defined budget frameworks.[5] The primary care led NHS became the vogue, much to the horror of many hospital colleagues who did not see GPs as being sufficiently knowledgeable about different speciality areas. But GPs, many of whom were in direct control of much of the services delivered to their patients through fundholding, had a clearer role in the planning and delivery of health services.

A final critical development that was to shape health care services for the future was the Patient's Charter.[6] This put the patient in the role of the consumer of health services with rights that forced both the purchasers and the providers of health services to adhere to standards of quality of care around different areas including waiting times, standards of communication and access to care.

Current context for working as a GP

To return to the examples in the introduction to this chapter, much of what is described there is not core clinical work. However, it is all will be under the control and influence of the business owners, most if not all of whom will be general practitioners, namely the partners in the practice. The practice manager will be a key player and in recent years in some more innovative practices the practice manager has been a profit-sharing partner, but always there will be at least one GP. So what qualities would a GP need to be a successful partner in a small general practice business?

Clearly a GP needs to be a competent practising doctor. This is the core of the work they do and it influences the way patients and colleagues view them and therefore the practice. But to return to the example in the introduction they need to be able to:

- Understand the organisational arrangements necessary to run a business including telephones, opening hours, appointment arrangements, etc.
- Delegate tasks to others effectively, ensuring that they will be followed through

- Ensure that their staff are trained so that the service aspired to can be delivered
- Communicate clearly and politely with staff and patients
- Recruit, retain and develop staff so that they can contribute to high-standard service delivery in the practice
- Manage their time effectively
- Negotiate with others in their team and agree shared protocols and procedures for the practice.

This list is not exhaustive but it gives a range of management activities that GPs can expect to be involved with to a varying degree on a daily basis to ensure the smooth running of their practice. An important area that has not been touched on is the whole question of financial management, e.g. paying staff, underpinning practice development (both staff and premises) and ensuring that the GP partners receive appropriate remuneration for their efforts in their profit shares. The practice manager and the practice accountant are important players but responsibility for this cannot be totally passed over to these people as primary care services are funded in complicated and changing ways, which ultimately shape the services offered by practices, with increased profits associated with higher quality in performance at a clinical level.

Practice management supporting practice development

The principles of good practice management centre round clear policies, systems and procedures that are understood and signed up by all. At the heart of this, as with any organisation whether large or small, is the culture of the organisation, how it feels to be part of that organisation or receive the services of that organisation. In recent years there has been greater emphasis on the impact of practice management systems on the services offered by a practice. Being part of a small business and able to influence how the practice provides services and develops its services is one of the big attractions of being a GP. Some GPs go on to study for a Master in Business Administration (MBA) degree and develop specific interests in health care management and delivery as a means of building on the management experience they gain on top of their clinical expertise as a GP.

How can a GP shape their practice's development?

Answer – through leadership. The NHS Plan[7] laid out far-reaching changes across the NHS in an attempt to improve service delivery in health care for the twenty-first century. A strong theme throughout this White Paper was the need to develop leadership in both the management and clinical aspects of the work. Clearly in hospital trusts, as larger organisations, there is a greater distinction between clinical and non-clinical responsibilities. But general practice is, as we have discussed earlier, a small business, and hence GP partners are never going to be far away from managerial responsibilities and decisions in their day-to-day work.

The Department of Health has given further details on what it had in mind in its NHS Leadership Qualities Framework.[8] This framework groups leadership qualities under three headings: personal qualities, setting direction and delivering the service. Under personal qualities it lists self-belief, self-awareness, self-management, drive for improvement and personal integrity as the key characteristics of an effective leader. To be an effective leader calls on different qualities and skills at different times, depending on the situation and the people involved.[9]

Much has been written about leadership styles in various contexts across all aspects of our lives and the history of civilisation. Indeed it must be remembered that being a leader does not equate with being a good person nor to being liked. However, to be a leader it is important to understand the history and background of the circumstances where you are playing the leader's role and to learn from your experiences and the experiences of other leaders to do the job properly. Many times one hears of Churchill's leadership skills during the Second World War and how others have subsequently learnt from and applied these skills.

To study Churchill[10] and his leadership style is to restrict the interpretation of leadership to a very autocratic authoritarian approach, successful during the Second World War, but not with the outbreak of peace. Pettinger[11] describes a spectrum of leadership styles with autocratic leadership at one end and democratic at the other. In between comes consultative leadership. Clearly different situations demand different leadership styles from the crisis where immediate action is required for helping the practice team, maybe with patient participation, develop practice facilities such as the appointment system. The skill will come in being able to switch from one leadership style to another, or to have the self-awareness to know that a particular situation demands the leadership skills of another member of your team.

In the late twentieth century there was growing interest and research into what makes organisations successful and the best ways that those organisations can maximise the full potential of the people working for them. Senge,[12] in his book *The Fifth Discipline,* describes what he calls the learning organisation – an organisation that is alive, always growing, changing and reviewing its work in its particular context and in line with current pressures and initiatives of change. The leaders working in such organisations are described as designers, stewards and teachers.

How can a practice become a learning organisation?

For a practice in primary care to be a learning organisation the leaders or partners need not only ensure that the necessary management and financial arrangements are in place as described above, but they also need to understand changes in policy and organisational arrangements in the health service and have a vision for how they want themselves and their practice to move forward. Such planning will include both clinical and non-clinical challenges and will require the ability to be able to handle the uncertainty of a developing situation and to be able to take decisions in an informed way, weighing up and balancing risk accordingly.

GPs as part of a leadership team in a practice will need to ensure that their practice team is developing the necessary knowledge and skills to be able to deliver the vision. To do this effectively GPs need to be able to understand how to motivate people to take on new ideas and change. They need to understand how adults learn[13] and how to harness that learning into practice. In primary care over recent years there has been a big drive to introduce annual appraisal for everyone in the practice team and for this to be the cornerstone of individual and practice development.

Recent public enquiries[14] into health service tragedies has criticised the robustness of appraisal systems to identify poor performance and has sighted individual and team governance as being key to quality performance across the NHS. Those in leadership roles in any practice in primary care will need to take responsibility to ensure that all aspects of the work done in the practice and of the care offered to patients are within the terms defined under *Good Medical Practice*.[15]

How can a GP ensure to be a trusted clinician and manager?

A principal factor recognised by the medical profession and Department of Health in promoting quality in primary care is the support and governance from peers and colleagues. Fewer GPs work in single-handed practices nowadays as it has become increasingly difficult to run an efficient practice offering a wide range of quality services as a single-handed GP. It is not impossible, however, and many single-handed practices offer the much desired continuity of care to patients as happens when there is only one doctor to deliver the services.

Whether a GP is single-handed or part of a 10-partner practice, seeking out support and supervision on his or her practice is an essential ingredient to practising safely and growing as a clinician and professional. That support could be in the form of mentorship (the support from a wise and trusted friend), which is widely associated with success at work and in life in general.[16] The nursing profession has long embraced mentoring as a key aspect of professional development, using it as a means of offering support and encouraging reflective practice.[17] An alternative model is that of clinical supervision[18] whereby a supervisor works with a practitioner, helping him or her to interpret the complexity of situations through skilled questioning and conversation.

Summary

A doctor working as a GP in a primary care practice needs to be a competent clinician and able to understand and provide leadership for the development planning, business management and human resources side of running a practice. In order to do this a GP needs to be able to work with his or her partners as a team player and to communicate with, support and develop the others in the practice through demonstrating clear vision, purpose and direction with all aspects of practice management.

References

1 Leathard A (1997) Interprofessional developments in Britain: an overview. In: Leathard (ed.) *Going Interprofessional: Working Together for Health and Welfare*. London: Routledge.
2 Pietroni P (1997) Interprofessional teamwork: its history and development in hospital, general practice and community care. In: Leathard (ed.) *Going Interprofessional: Working Together for Health and Welfare*. London: Routledge.
3 Beveridge Report (1942) *Interdepartmental Committee on Social Insurance and Allied Services*. London: HMSO.
4 Griffiths R (1983) *NHS Management Inquiry*. London: HMSO.
5 Department of Health (1991) *The Health of the Nation*. London: HMSO.
6 Department of Health (1992) *Patient's Charter*. London: HMSO.
7 Department of Health (2000) *The NHS Plan: A Plan for Investment, a Plan for Reform*. London: DoH.
8 Department of Health (2006) http://www.nhsleadershipqualities.nhs.uk/
9 Firth-Cozens J (2006) Leadership and the quality of healthcare. In: Cox, King, Hutchinson and McAvoy (eds) *Understanding Doctors' Performance*. Oxford: Radcliffe.
10 Roberts A (2003) *Hitler and Churchill: Secrets of Leadership*. London: Phoenix.
11 Pettiger R (1997) *Introduction to Management*. London: MacMillan.
12 Senge P (2006) *The Fifth Discipline: The Art and Practice of the Learning Organisation*. London: Random House.

13 Brookfield S (1986) Understanding how adults learn. *Understanding and Facilitating Adult Learning.* Buckingham: Open University Press.

14 Smith J (2004) *Safeguarding Patients: Learning Lessons From the Past, Proposals for the Future.* London: The Stationery Office.

15 General Medical Council (2006) *Good Medical Practice.* London: General Medical Council.

16 Morton-Cooper A, Palmer A (2000) *Mentorship, Preceptorship and Clinical Supervision.* London: Blackwell.

17 Schon D (1983) *The Reflective Practitioner: How Professionals Think in Action.* London: Temple Smith.

18 Burton J, Launer J (2003) Primary care and the need for clinical supervision and support. In: Burton and Launer (eds) *Supervision and Support in Primary Care.* Oxford: Radcliffe.

Chapter 18 **Towards retirement**

Roger May

Introduction

Many, if not most people at work dream of their retirement ... all that leisure ... all that pleasure ... all that freedom. As the great day draws nearer the prospect may become more scary ... 'How will we manage?' ... Where shall we live? ... What shall we actually do? Maybe, even, how will we get on cooped up together all day long? (This and following sections assume the existence of a spouse or life partner – those on their own are asked to please forbear.)

This chapter sets out to give you some things to think about even now that may better prepare you for your retirement. It aims to help you decide:

- *Why* retire?
- *When* should you retire?
- *What* should your retirement look like?
- *How* should you prepare for it?

The chapter begins by inviting you to consider your own particular *value system* and *emotional make up* and the needs they produce that you will have to satisfy in order to maintain a fulfilling retirement. Next, we look at the *balance sheet* of retirement, the gains and the losses that retirement brings. More practical thoughts follow including *fiscal considerations* and some thoughts on the *choices of activities* that await you. Then come two sections covering the *unpredictability of your own life* and the *influence of other people* on your proposals. The chapter draws towards its close with a section entitled '*What should you think about now?*' and it finishes with a short *summary*.

Attitudes, beliefs and feelings

Why, really, did you become a doctor? Was it for status? Money? Security? To please your parents? Or was there a true sense of vocation? To a greater

---

Choosing General Practice: Your Career Guide. Edited by Anne Hastie and Anne Stephenson. © 2008 Blackwell Publishing, ISBN: 978-1-4501-7070-3.

or lesser extent the decision reflected the value base, the belief system that you held at that time. That system, however modified by the passing of the years, will influence the decisions around your retirement, consciously or subconsciously. So too will your emotional make up. It is said that there are seven basic emotional needs that drive us all. They are the need for love and security, for praise and recognition, for challenge and responsibility and, lastly, the need for new experiences. The proportion of each that affects us varies from person to person and to a degree within the same individual at different times. Some of these needs will be met partially or fully by our religion, our hobbies or within our personal relationships but for all of us a significant proportion will be satisfied in our daily work. The question therefore is: *how will my emotional needs be met in my retirement?*

Thinking about that question will bring to the surface some of your basic attitudes and highlight several questions. For example, are we on this earth to serve our own needs exclusively or those of other people also? Is it alright to set aside one's experience, skills, knowledge and expertise of our own volition or should one seek to continue to use all of one's talents as long as possible? Does the completion of, say, 30 years as a GP somehow entitle one to put one's feet up for the rest of one's life? We each have to find the answers to these and similar questions for ourselves. We shall, of course, ask the opinion of those who we love and trust and who know us best but wise counsellors will remind you that the only person who can have the final say is you. Maybe the best place to start is to think about whether one wants to continue an active professional role to some extent. If the answer to that seems to be in the affirmative then spend a while working out why exactly that might be. Is it for financial reasons? Are you merely seeking to continue to meet your own emotional needs in the way most familiar to you? Is it a need to be needed perhaps? May be it is even something about exercising control or power? Or are you clear that carrying on working in some way reflects your *genuine* values and beliefs?

The retirement balance sheet

As you think about retirement you may find it helpful to draw up a balance sheet, listing the perceived gains and losses of your plans.

Some of the losses have already been alluded to in the preceding section. Inevitably income will decline, although, not necessarily your standard of living. For better or worse you will lose the close daily contacts with partners, staff and patients. The resulting loss of fellowship may be keenly felt. Less tangible but equally important for many is the loss of structure to one's life, the loss of routine. More telling still maybe the loss of self-worth, most of us enjoy our daily ration of hearing ourselves called 'doctor' and receiving some respect for our wisdom and position in society. Feeling useful and feeling valued are important to us all.

What of the gains? There are two obvious 'biggies' – the reduction of stress and the gaining of time. Giving up the daily grind, the hassle, the pressure, the emotional and physical demands will be in the front of one's mind. Life will still have its problems but far, far less. Secondly, the issue of time. Time to take things at a more leisurely pace. Time indeed for more leisure. Time to think, to relax, to read and perhaps to write. Time to pursue those hobbies and pastimes. Time perhaps to do good works. Time to see friends, to travel, to take up new interests and to develop old ones. Time to breathe and to just be. Bliss!

Or is it? Time to do a greater share of the domestic chores, the weekly shop, those countless tasks in home and garden. Time to visit that tiresome old aunt, and no excuse not to. And, for those in a close personal relationship, much more time to spend with that relative stranger with whom one has somehow passed the last ever so many years before 'I married him for better or for worse but not for lunch!'

More seriously there may well be other real gains for you. Relatively minor things like the release from the need to keep up to date and from the feelings of guilt that accompany those unopened medical journals. You may find it a relief not to have to spend time almost exclusively in the company of other doctors. Major things too, such as the ability to move to new surroundings, do a new degree or even take up another profession. Writing this side of the balance sheet will help you to begin to consider the almost frightening number of choices that will lie before you. We shall return to some of these thoughts in the section marked 'Activities'.

Fiscal considerations

When we are starting a job few of us give very much thought to what our income will be in retirement but as the big day draws near the question in the front of our minds is likely to be *'Will I have enough to see me through?'* It is perhaps a question worth some thought earlier rather than later. Here are some facts.

1 In 2004/2005 the average UK GP in partnership earned in excess of £80,000.
2 Over the years GP income has kept up with inflation fairly well.
3 Arguably the BMA is one of the world's strongest unions.
4 The earnings of most GP partners rise rapidly over the first few years and then, in real terms, stay fairly level for the rest of their career.
5 At the time of writing the NHS pension scheme is under review but it will certainly continue to provide a substantial income in retirement

for all who contribute through a working life of normal duration. Also, GPs will continue to benefit from a particularly flexible package and a substantial lump sum when they finish work.

6 GPs will also be entitled to the normal State pension.

The problem for all of us is the declining value of money. Over the last 10 years inflation has averaged approximately 2.6% per annum but it can get out of control. In 1975 it was over 24% and as recently as 1990 it was well over 9%. Since 1983 the cost of most things has roughly doubled. When thinking about retirement income one has to project not only to the day one finishes work but through to one's death and even possibly beyond that, to the death of one's spouse.

The question therefore is: '*Should I be saving for retirement in addition to my basic pension and if so how?*' For many the immediate answer is 'a chance would be a fine thing!' However, there does come a time when expenses die down and real choices as to how to use one's money arise. What should you do?

Here are some thoughts:

1 Have a close look at the NHS pension scheme and its options first. The BMA website is a good place to start.

2 Take professional advice from a good accountant and a good investment broker. If you contemplate using insurance try to use a broker who is independent and not on commission from a particular firm.

3 Insurance policies that promise huge payouts in the distant future do not always come up to scratch. Even if the company performs well remember that what looks like enough to buy a mansion in Bermuda now will probably only buy a push bike by the time you get to it in 20 years time!

4 Many so-called savings accounts do very little more than keep up with inflation.

5 Over the years house prices and therefore values have kept ahead of inflation. The UK average in 1983 was under £32,000 and in 2006 over £190,000. For many people moving up the scale with a view to down-sizing in later years has proved rewarding in the past.

6 Second homes have an obvious attraction but they bring substantial running costs and they are liable to capital gains tax on sale.

7 Investing in antiques, art, stamps, wine and so on demands real expertise. The people who make most money from them are the dealers!

Activities

For many the sentence 'I am retiring ....' is completed by the words '... and moving to Margate/Scotland/Costa Fortune'. A mistake. Consider first what you want to *do* in retirement then where you want to do it.

As mentioned before the first question is *whether or not to continue to work* in some way. There are lots of options in your field – a full-time GP but without the responsibilities of partnership; part-time GP, locum; emergency work, etc. You will need to consider whether it will be in your old practice or in pastures new. If the latter, locally or further afield? How many hours in the day? How many days a week? And for how many years?

The fact is that many GPs simply cannot face life without some clinical contact. Others wish to remain associated with the profession but are happy to give up seeing patients. For them work with the Local Medical Committee (LMC) or in health management may fit the bill. Others will develop a post with an insurance company, in medical education or in a field of special interest such as sports medicine or acupuncture, for example.

On the other hand some people are able to give up work entirely and without regret. What do they do with themselves? Assuming good health and no other major commitments such as being a carer their choices fall largely into four areas:

1 Volunteering
2 Learning
3 Sports and hobbies
4 Pastimes.

The United Kingdom is unique in the opportunities that are available for voluntary work. Charities of all kinds cry out for helpers, board members, trustees and chairmen. Churches, Temples and Synagogues rely heavily on support from their members. So too do the National Trust, the Red Cross, the Citizens Advice Bureau, the Samaritans, Alcohol Advisory Groups, local and national parties and countless other organisations. Some, such as Rotary, Soroptimists and the Masons combine good works with fellowship.

Good doctors are lifelong learners and retirement will not change that although the focus of study may change. Time then to follow up that research or branch out into something new from archaeology or art appreciation to zoology or Zoroastrianism. You could sign up for the Open University or take a master's degree. Local council day and evening classes abound and in many areas the University of the Third Age and the Workers Education Association are active. Again the possibilities are endless.

Most of us have some suitable sporting activity or pursue a hobby that we would wish to take into retirement. The best keep us fit in mind or body and provide social contact. Some, such as collecting, making jewellery or running an allotment, may even be financially profitable.

Pastimes on the other hand, although pleasurable, bring little demonstrable benefit apart from their immediate pleasure. Perhaps daytime television, surfing the net and reading cheap novels fall into this category. But why not look forward to them too?

There are, of course, some activities that do not sit comfortably within one of the four rather arbitrary areas used above. Travel comes to mind, so too does the appreciation of music and music making.

It would seem that those who are happiest in retirement are those who construct a portfolio of things to do, perhaps choosing at least one from each of the categories and maybe some that reach across them.

Here then are the questions that arise from this section:

Would it be wise to begin to think about what your set of retirement activities, your portfolio, might look like and whether there are things that you can do at this time in preparation?

Answer that and you will be able to quickly determine whether Margate is the right place for you!

Yourself

Everybody's life is unpredictable, even yours. For example new personal relationships, divorce, even widowhood may intervene. Other calamities may befall you – illness or serious injury, addiction to alcohol, drugs or gambling, even, heaven forbid, medical disgrace. For all of these reasons planning for retirement can, at best, only ever be tentative.

Health, however, is a different matter. *Maintaining fitness* is something that we can all attend to straight away. Lucky the person who escapes all the penalties of the ageing process, be it declining energy and physical strength, maybe lessening mobility or memory, some deafness perhaps or even failing sight. Until those days dawn it behoves us all to do what we can to keep our bodies in shape, the non-medical bits of our brain alert and our spiritual life nourished. Easier said than done for busy GPs. Incidentally you may wish to consider *health insurance* at this stage too. Once one does finally leave the NHS and one's contacts fall away you may find it reassuring to know that you can call on someone else to pay for your treatment when it becomes a necessity.

Other people

When contemplating retirement there are two considerations to be made under this heading.

Firstly, *what duties and obligations will be placed upon my time by others?* Ageing parents are the most obvious example. For most of us there comes a time when our relationship changes from dependent child through mature adult to one of overseer, guardian or carer. Their increasing physical frailty, perhaps decreasing mobility, maybe mental impairment, could well place demands upon you. For some similar challenges arise because of a child, sibling or other close relative who has special needs. Sometimes of course it is one's own life partner who presents similar problems that have to be faced. For all of us the unpredictability of such matters makes planning ahead more difficult. If all this sounds rather gloomy it should be said that many of us find great joy in supporting our families, especially lending a hand with the grandchildren for instance. Indeed, for many retirees this may become their chief activity and their chief pleasure.

The second consideration centres around *the depth of relationship that one would wish to maintain with all the other people in one's life when the time commitments reduce.* The emotional closeness and physical proximity of one's children is the most obvious example. Many retirees make the decision to move nearer to their children – a move that needs to be thought through most carefully. Who else will you keep in touch with? You may well find that those with whom you had daily contact at work are now consumed by new relationships. Many whom you regarded as friends in that context may now prove to have been ships that passed in the night. *The cultivation of friendships,* especially friendships beyond medicine, is something that you may wish to pay attention to right now.

What should you think about now?

This chapter opened by suggesting that preparation for retirement might focus on the reasons for retiring, when to retire, what you wish to do in retirement and how best to prepare for it. Many do find that the prospect of life without work is a surprisingly daunting prospect and choose to postpone it or take up the option of part-time employment for a while. Sooner or later however most of us reach the big R and this section sets out the questions that you might reasonably ask yourself *right now* in preparation. It starts with the most difficult:

1 What are the things about work that meet my emotional needs and match my personal value base that I shall have to meet in some other ways in retirement?

2 What does my own retirement balance sheet look like – the gains and the losses?

3 Do I fully understand the NHS pension scheme, and the options that it offers me?

4 Am I satisfied that I am receiving sound and truly independent financial advice?

5 What measures should I be taking now to guard against inflation and the financial effects of possible illness or accident?

6 What are likely to be my unavoidable obligations in retirement and how will they constrain the pattern of activities that I would wish to pursue?

7 What voluntary work, sports, hobbies and pastimes can I develop now to take forward into retirement?

8 Am I thinking widely enough when I contemplate other activities that I might pursue?

9 Am I taking care to develop friendships and social connections, especially non-medical ones that I shall be able to take on into retirement?

10 Am I doing everything possible to maintain my fitness?

And, *most importantly*, for those of us blessed with a close personal relationship:

11 How does all of this fit in with the needs and wishes of my life partner?

Summary

This chapter invites you to begin to think about life after work sooner rather than later. It poses a series of questions that may help you to determine whether you should retire and if so when. It invites you to think about what your retirement might look like and it contains some prompts to help you to prepare for it.

In conclusion it might be worth reminding you that the most common response from retirees as to how they are managing is 'I cannot imagine how I ever had time to go to work'. Many joys await you.

Index